CORONARY ANGIOSCOPY

by

Yasumi Uchida, MD

President, Japan Foundation of Cardiovascular Research
Professor, Clinical Physiology and Cardiovascular Center
Toho University Hospital at Sakura
Sakura, Japan

FUTURA

Futura Publishing Company, Inc.
Armonk, NY

Library of Congress Cataloging-in-Publication Data

Uchida, Yasumi.
  Coronary angioscopy / by Yasumi Uchida.
     p. ; cm.
  Includes bibliographical references and index.
  ISBN 0-87993-478-6
  1. Angioscopy. 2. Coronary heart disease—Diagnosis. I. Title.
  [DNLM: 1. Angioscopy. 2. Coronary Disease—diagnosis. WG 300 U105c 2001]
RC691.6.A53 U25 2001

                                                                    00-052153

Copyright 2001
Futura Publishing Company, Inc.

Published by
Futura Publishing Company, Inc.
135 Bedford Road
Armonk, NY 10504

LC #: 00-052153
ISBN #: 0-87993-478-6

To

Akiko, Yuuko, Harkuko, Yasuto,

and all my co-workers

Preface

In 1925, Dr. Kussmal in Germany devised a metallic tube with an attached lens inside for observation of the interior of stomach. This was the first clinically applied endoluminal scope (endoscope). However, since it was rigid, introducing it through the mouth and into the stomach was a great burden on patients.

On August 31, 1945, a big storm attacked the Kanto district of Japan. Trains were stopped for several hours due to the storm, and Dr. T. Uji, a surgeon at Tokyo University, and Mr. M. Sugiura of Olympus Company happened to meet on the train. A concept of a new endoscope was discussed, which would be the start of the development of the endoscope in Japan.

In December 1949, in collaboration with M. Fukaomi and M. Maruyama, they developed a flexible gastroscope 12 mm in diameter with film and an illumination source in the distal-most tip. Anesthetized dogs were successfully examined with this endoscope.

T. Sakamoto used this endoscope for the first time as a gastroscope. The flexible gastroscope thus developed has been the basic structure for the bronchoscope, the cystoscope, etc.

Several years later, this gastroscope was replaced by a fiberscope that was more flexible and more easily manipulated. Fiberscopes are now widely used in the diagnosis and treatment not only of disorders and diseases of the digestive tract but they are also an essential tool in the diagnosis and treatment of disorders and diseases of the respiratory and urogenital tracts.

Although the endoscope was clinically applied to the peripheral artery during surgery by S.M. Greenstone, many years passed until percutaneous transluminal coronary angioscopy was performed. This was due to the difficulty in the displacement of blood in the artery and the need for a thinner, more flexible endoscope.

With the anticipation of clinical application, we (Y. Uchida and members of Olympus Co.) began to develop a new fiberscope for coronary use in 1976. Thrombosis and thrombolysis in the removed human coronary artery and the changes induced by balloon angioplasty were successfully observed using this endoscope in 1984.

Meanwhile, J.R. Spears reported percutaneous transluminal application of the fiberscope for observation of the coronary artery. He observed coronary ostia by the use of a broncoscope (1983). Also, coronary arterial changes were observed mainly intraoperatively by F. Litback (1985), F. Homebach (1986), T.A. Sanborn (1986), C.T. Sherman (1985), T. Vent (1987), etc.

Using fiberscopes especially designed for coronary use, the author observed percutaneously the proximal to distal coronary segments in patients with ischemic heart disease (1984, 1987). Observation of plaque disruption and thrombi in acute coronary syndromes was performed by V.H. Holer (1988), K. Mizuno (1991), P. den Heijer (1994), P.J. de Feyter (1995), J.A. Silva (1995), T. Thieme (1996), S. Waxman (1997), and others. Evaluation of coronary interventions by plain old balloon angioplasty (POBA) was performed by M.A. Sassour (1993), the author (1984), P. den Heijer (1994) and A. Itoh (1995). Coronary intervention by laser was evaluated by the author (1987), F. Nakamura (1992), and A. Itoh (1993), and evaluation of coronary interventions by directional coronary atherectomy (DCA), stent, and cutting balloon were carried out by many investigators.

Application of percutaneous coronary angioscopy was extended to diagnosis of Kawasaki disease by T. Ishikawa, my colleague, (1991) and for observation of coronary artery bypass grafting (CABG) by the author (1994).

Meanwhile, an angioscope of the monorail type without a balloon was devised by the author (1989), one with a balloon by Baxter Co., and a 3-channel angioscopy balloon catheter by the author (1994). Fiberscopes for coronary use are now reduced in an outer diameter down to 1 F. Thus, percutaneous angioscopy is now routinely performed at several institutions for examination of underlying mechanisms of acute coronary syndromes, for selection of therapeutic modalities, for evaluation of medical, interventional, and surgical therapies, and for prediction of acute coronary syndromes.

In 1999, dye image coronary angioscopy was established by us based on animal experiments for identification of endothelial damage. Fluorescent image coronary angioscopy was also performed clinically by the author (1999).

These new techniques may yield more detailed information on composition and metabolism of coronary plaques. Angioscope-guided transcatheter interventions that were applied to peripheral vessel disease (1992) may also be applied to the coronary artery in the near future. Currently, angioscopes for coronary use contain more than 8000 glass or silica fibers that may give us much more improved images of coronary luminal changes. Angiomicroscopy, which enables evaluation of vascular changes at the cellular level, was applied to peripheral vessels (1995), and may also be applied to the coronary artery when it becomes flexible.

Observation of coronary microvessels is beyond conventional angioscopy. One possible approach for observation of coronary microvessels is their observation from inside of the cardiac chambers.

In 1912, Dr. von Rhea and Walker observed the interior of the heart during thoracotomy. In 1922, D.S. Allen, and in 1944, D.E. Harken also observed the interior of the heart during thoracotomy in animals. In 1948, by using a rigid endoscope, S. Sakakibara and his colleagues observed the interior of the right heart during open heart surgery. This may be the first observation of the interior of the heart in humans. However, many years passed before percutaneous cardioscopy was performed for observation of the interior of the beating heart in patients due to lack of a thin fiberscope and effective equipment for displacement of blood.

In 1988, the author successfully observed percutaneously the right and left ventricles from inside using a thin fiberscope incorporated in a guiding balloon catheter in anesthetized dogs, and it was applied in patients with heart disease in 1988. Application of this "cardioscopy" was extended to dilated cardiomyopathy, myocarditis, hypertrophic cardiomyopathy, and ischemic heart disease, and for evaluation of drugs on subendocardial microcirculation (1995).

In addition, cardioscope-guided endomyocardial biopsy has been established (1990). Now, dye image and fluorescent image cardioscopy are being clinically attempted. Cardioscope-guided intramyocardial and intrapericardial drug administration was recently started.

In 1996, intracardiac ultrasonography (ICUS) was also established and it is routinely used clinically for evaluation of cardiac chambers and valves. Combined use of cardioscopy and ICUS gives us much more information on cardiac wall architecture.

All angioscopic and cardioscopic images included in this book were obtained either by myself or by our colleagues under my supervision at Toho University Hospital at Sakura, Tokyo University, Funabashi-Futawa Hospital, and Narita Red Cross Hospital.

On April 1, 2000, the Japanese Association for Cardioangioscopy was founded based on 13 years of preceding activities using cardioangioscopy. Cardioangioscopy is now supported by the national health insurance in Japan.

Many years have passed since I started to establish coronary angioscopy and cardioscopy. I express sincere gratitude to Olympus Co., members of the Japan Foundation of Cardiovascular Research, and co-workers for their cooperation for many years. I express sincere gratitude to my wife, Akiko, for her warm encouragement and love. Also, I would also like to thank Futura Publishing Company for giving me the opportunity to publish this book.

Yasumi Uchida, MD

Members of Japan Foundation of Cardiovascular Research

Colleagues

1. **Toho University Hospital at Sakura**
   Cardiovascular Center
   Hidefumi Ohsawa, MD
   Hirobumi Noike, MD
   Keiichi Tokuhiro, MD
   Masahito Kanai, MD
   Masaki Yoshinuma, MD
   Kaneyuki Aoyagi, MD
   Pathology
   Noriaki Kameda, MD

   Takashi Sakurai, MD
   Kunio Yoshinaga, MD
   Takashi Uchi, MD
   Kouichi Kawamura, MD
   Takeshi Hitsumoto, MD

   Keishi Hiruta, MD

2. **Narita Red Cross Hospital**
   Cardiology
   Yoshiharu Fujimori, MD
   Kuniko Terasawa, MD

   Hiroshi Morio, MD
   Masaaki Ozegawa, MD

3. **Tokyo University**
   Cardiology
   Toshihiro Morita, MD
   Nephrology
   Haruko Uchida, PhD

   Fumitaka Nakamura, MD

   Kenjiro Kimura, MD

4. **Medical Center of Japanese Red Cross**
   Cardiology
   Takanobu Tomaru, MD

5. **Funabashi-Futawa Hospital**
   Cardiology
   Tomomitsu Ohshima, MD
   Satoru Morizuki, MD
   Masami Ishikawa, MD

   Jyunichi Hirose, MD
   Kazuko Kawamura, MD

Contents

PART I

Clinical Application of Percutaneous Coronary Angioscopy

Chapter 1

History of Coronary Angioscopy:

An Overview of the Literature

Endoscopes used for observation of the interior of the vessels are called angioscopes. Currently, only fiberscopes are clinically used for angioscopy. Therefore, fiberscopes alone or those incorporated into a guiding catheter are called angioscopes. An angioscopy system is composed of an angioscope, an illumination source, a recording system (cine camera, video recorder with either tape or disc), a monitor, and an injector.

Thus far, many articles on coronary plaque and thrombus characterization, selection of therapeutic modalities, evaluation of medical, interventional, and surgical therapies, and prognosis have been reported and are listed here.

Animal Experiments

Litvack F, Grundfest WS, Lee ME, Carroll RM, Foran R, Chaux A, Berci G, Rose HB, Matroff JM, Forrester JS: Angioscopic visualization of blood vessel interior in animals and humans. Clin Cardiol 8:65–70, 1985.

Tomaru T, Uchida Y, Kato A, Sonoki H, Sugimoto T: Experimental canine arterial thrombus formation and thrombolysis. Am Heart J 114:63–70, 1987.

Uchida Y, Nakamura F, Tomaru T, Sonoki H, Sugimoto T: Fiberoptic observation of blood flow through stenotic artery: A rheological mechanism of thrombosis. Am Heart J 118:1504–1506, 1987.

Removed Human Coronary Artery

Uchida Y, Tomaru T, Sumino S, Kato A, Sugimoto T: Fiberoptic observation of thrombosis and thrombolysis in isolated human coronary artery. Am Heart J 112:694–696, 1986.

Uchida Y, Kanai M, Takeuchi K, Kameda N, Hiruta K,

Uchida H, Uchida Y: Angioscopic characteristics of vulnerable coronary plaque and its pathological correlations. Coronary 16:302–313, 1999.

During Cardiac Surgery

Spears JR, Marais HJ, Serur J, Pomerantzeff O, Geyer DRP, Sipzener RS, Weintraub R, Thurer R, Paulin S, Gerstin R, Grossman W: In vivo angioscopy. J Am Coll Cardiol 1:1311–1314, 1983.

Litvack F, Grundfest WS, Lee ME, Carroll RM, Foran R, Chaux A, Berci G, Rose HB, Matroff JM, Forrester JS: Angioscopic visualization of blood vessel interior in animals and humans. Clin Cardiol 8:65–70, 1985.

Sanborn TA, Rygaard JA, Westbrook BM, Lazar HL, McCormick JR, Roberts AJ, Madroff I: Intraoperative angioscopy of saphenous vein and coronary arteries. Thorac Cardiovasc Surg 91:339–343, 1986.

Hombach V, Hoeher M, Hannekum A, Hugel W, Buran B, Hoeppe HW, Hirche H: Erste klinische Erfarlungen mit der Koronarendoskopie. Deut Medi Wochen 30:1135–1140, 1986.

Sherman CT, Litvak F, Grundfest W, Lee M, Hickey A, Chaux A, Kass R, Blanche C, Matroff J, Morgenstein L, Ganz W, Swan HJC, Forrester J: Coronary angioscopy in patients with unstable angina pectoris. N Engl J Med 315:919–919, 1986.

Percutaneous Coronary Angioscopy

Plaque Characterization

Spears JR, Spokojny AM, Marais HJ: Coronary angioscopy during cardiac catheterization. J Am Coll Cardiol 6:93–97, 1985.

Uchida Y, Tomaru T, Nakamura F, Furuse A, Fujimori Y: Percutaneous coronary angioscopy in patients with ischemic heart disease. Am Heart J 114:1216–1222, 1987.

Kuwaki K, Inoue K, Ueda K, Shirai T, Ochiai H: Percutaneous transluminal coronary angioscopy during cardiac catheterization. Circulation 76:IV-185, 1987 (abstract).

Hoeher M, Homback V, Hoepp HW, Hilger HH: Percutaneous coronary angioscopy during cardiac catheterization. J Am Coll Cardiol 11:65A, 1988 (abstract).

Uchida Y: Percutaneous coronary angioscopy by means of a fiberscope with steerable guidewire. Am Heart J 117:1153–1155, 1989.

Uchida Y: Percutaneous cardiovascular angioscopy. In: Lasers in Cardiovascular Medicine and Surgery. Abela G (ed). Kluwer Academic Publishers, Boston, MA, 1989, pp 399–410.

Mizuno K, Miyamoto A, Satomura K, Kurita A, Arai T, Sakurada M, Yanagida S, Nakamura H: Angioscopic coronary macromorphology in patients with acute coronary syndromes. Lancet 337:809–812, 1991.

Ishikawa H, Uchida Y: Angioscopic features of coronary artery in Kawasaki disease. Proceedings of 4th International Kawasaki Disease Conference, pp 20–22, 1991.

Uchida Y, Hirose J, Fujimori Y, Oshima T: Percutaneous coronary angioscopy. Jpn Heart J 33:271–294, 1992.

den Heijer P, Foley DP, Escaned J, Hillege HL, Serruys P, Lie KI: Angioscopic versus angiographic detection of intimal dissection and intracoronary thrombus. J Am Coll Cardiol 24:649–654, 1994.

Silva JA, Escobar A, Collins TJ, Ramee SR, White CJ: Unstable angina: A comparison of angioscopic findings between diabetic and nondiabetic patients. Circulation 92:1731–1736, 1995.

Itoh A, Miyazaki S, Nonogi H, Daikoku S, Haze K: Angioscopic prediction of successful dilatation and of restenosis in percutaneous transluminal coronary angioplasty. Circulation 91:1389–1396, 1995.

Thieme T, Wernicke KD, Meyer R, Brandenstein E, Habedank D, Hinz A, Felix S, Baumann G, Kleber FX: Angioscopic evaluation of atherosclerotic plaques: Validation by histomorphologic analysis and association with stable and unstable coronary syndromes. JACC 28:1–6, 1996.

Waxman S, Mittleman MA, Zarich SW, Fitzpatrick PI, Lewis SM, Leeman DE, Shubrooks SJ Jr, Snyder JT, Muller JE, Nesto RW: Angioscopic assessment of coronary lesions underlying thrombus. Am J Cardiol 79:1106–1109, 1997.

Hombach V, Hoeler M, Koches M, Eggeling T, Schmidt A, Hoep HW, Hilger HH: Pathophysiology of unstable angina pectoris: Correlations with coronary angioscopic imaging. Eur Heart J 9:40–45, 1998.

Comparison with Intravascular Ultrasound (IVUS)

Feyter PJ, Ozaki Y, Baptista J, Escaned J, DiMario C, de Jaegere PPT, Serruys P, Roeland JRTC: Ischemia-related lesion characteristics in patients with stable or unstable angina: A study with intracoronary angioscopy and ultrasound. Circulation 92:1408–1413, 1995.

Dye Image Coronary Angioscopy

Fujimori Y, Morio H, Terasawa K, Matsuo T, Ozegawa M, Uchida Y: Damages of coronary endothelial cells are easily caused even by floppy guidewire: In vivo staining angioscopic study. J Am Coll Cardiol 33(Suppl A):67A, 1999 (abstract).

Fujimori Y, Terasawa K, Yamada K, Hasegawa O, Matsuo T, Ozegawa T, Uchida Y: Angioscopic evaluation of coronary endothelial lesions by staining with Evans blue in patients with acute myocardial infarction. J Am Coll Cardiol 33(Suppl A):67A, 1999 (abstract).

Fujimori Y, Morio H, Terasawa K, Hasegawa O, Matsuo T, Ozegawa M, Uchida Y: Characteristics of the culprit coronary lesions and estimation of the interventional treatments in patients with acute myocardial infarction by coronary angioscopy. J Am Coll Cardiol 33(Suppl A):64A, 1999 (abstract).

Morio H, Fujimori Y, Terasawa K, Matsuo T, Ozegawa M, Uchida Y: Evaluation of culprit coronary lesions for unstable angina pectoris by angioscopy. Jpn Circulat J 63(Suppl I):259, 1999 (abstract).

Terasawa K, Fujimori Y, Morio H, Yamada K, Matsuo T, Ozegawa M, Uchida Y: Evaluation of coronary endothelial cell damages caused by PTCA guidewire: In vivo dye staining angioscopy. J Jpn Coll Angiol 40:159–164, 2000.

Fluorescence Image Coronary Angioscopy

Uchida Y, Ohsawa H, Takeuchi K: Fluorescence coronary angioscopy. Jpn Circulat 63(Suppl I):310, 1999 (abstract).

During Interventions

Uchida Y, Tomaru T, Sugimoto T: Angioscopic observation of coronary luminal changes induced by PTCA. Proceedings of Jpn Coll Angiol, p 50, 1984 (abstract).

Uchida Y. Hasegawa K, Kawamura K, Shibuya I: Angioscopic observation of the coronary luminal changes induced by percutaneous transluminal coronary angioplasty. Am Heart J 117:769–776, 1989.

Ramee SR, White JC, Mesa JE, Murgo JP: Percutaneous angioscopy during coronary angioplasty using a steerable microangioscope. J Am Coll Cardiol 17:100–105, 1991.

Nakamura F, Kvasnicka J, Uchida Y, Geschwind HJ: Percutaneous angioscopic evaluation of luminal changes induced by excimer laser angioplasty. Am Heart J 124:1467–1472, 1992.

Itoh A, Miyazaki S, Nonogi H, Ozono K, Daikoku S, Saito K, Goto Y, Haze K: Angioscopic and intravascular ultrasound imagings before and after percutaneous Holmium-YAG laser coronary angioplasty. Am Heart J 125:556–558, 1993.

Sassower MA, Abela GS, Koch JM, Manzo KM, Friedl SE, Vivino PG, Nesto RW: Angioscopic evaluation of periprocedural abrupt closure after percutaneous coronary angioplasty. Am Heart J 126:444–450, 1993.

Ueda Y, Nanto S, Komamura K, Kodama K: Neointimal coverage of stents in human coronary arteries observed by angioscopy. J Am Coll Cardiol 23:341–346, 1994.

Tsukahara R, Hou M, Muramatsu M: Characteristics of culprit coronary plaques in chronic stage in patients with acute myocardial infarction. Coronary 15:145–150, 1998 (in Japanese).

Tsukahara R, Muramatsu T, Hou M, Inoue K, Akimoto T, Hirano K, Itoh S: The efficacy of direct stent in acute myocardial infarction and healing process evaluated by angioscopy and intravascular ultrasound. J Jpn Coll Angiol 39:17–22, 1999 (in Japanese).

Prognosis

Uchida Y, Nakamura F, Tomaru T, Morita T, Oshima T, Sasaki T, Morizuki S, Hirose J: Prediction of acute coronary syndromes by percutaneous coronary angioscopy in patients with stable angina pectoris. Am Heart J 130:195–203, 1995.

Ueda Y, Asakura M, Hirayama A, Kodama K: Intracoronary morphology of culprit lesions after reperfusion in acute myocardial infarction: Serial angioscopic observation. J Am Coll Cardiol 27:606–610, 1996.

Uchida Y: Angioscopic detection of vulnerable plaques and prediction of acute coronary syndromes. In: The Vulnerable Atherosclerotic Plaque: Understanding, Identification and Modification. Fuster V (ed). Futura Publishing Co, Armonk, NY, 1999, pp 111–129.

Medical Treatment

Uchida Y, Fujimori Y, Ohsawa H, Hirose J, et al: Angioscopic evaluation of the stabilizing effects of bezafibrate on coronary plaques. Coronary 16:293–301, 1999 (in Japanese).

Coronary Bypass Graft

Uchida Y, Fujimori Y, Hirose J, Oshima T: Percutaneous coronary angioscopy. Jpn Heart J 33:271–294, 1992.

Annex BH, Ajlini SC, Larkin TJ, O'Neil WW, Safian RD: Angioscopic guided interventions in a saphenous vein graft. Cathet Cardiovasc Diag 31:330–333, 1994.

Chapter 2

Coronary Angioscopes That Have Been Devised in Our Laboratories

Figs. 1–4 show angioscopes that have been developed in our laboratories in collaboration with Olympus Co., Tokyo, and Clinical Supply Co., Gifu, Japan.

In 1976, Y. Uchida and Olympus Co. developed a 10 F fiberscope. This was used for observation of the interior of the removed human coronary artery. Since it was too big, it was not used for percutaneous coronary angioscopy in patients but was used for observation of coronary bypass grafts during bypass surgery.

In 1977, in anticipation of clinical application, a 5 F fiberscope, 4000 px and 2-m long, was developed. This fiberscope was very flexible and its distal tip was smooth. After confirmation of its feasibility in dogs, it was first applied, in combination with a 9 F guiding catheter used for PTCA, for observation of the coronary artery from the proximal to the distal segments. The observed coronary luminal changes were recorded on a 16-mm color cine film (Fig. 1). This was probably the first fiberscope used to percutaneously observe the coronary artery in humans.

In subsequent years, in order to obtain coaxiality and effective blood displacement, 1.6 F and 2.7 F fiberscopes were developed. These fiberscopes were introduced deep into the coronary artery through an inner guiding catheter (Fig. 2A). This angioscopy system is still used in selected patients. A 5 F fiberscope with a central lumen that allows a 0.018-inch guidewire to pass through was also developed (Fig. 2B). However, this angioscopy system was not used clinically because of insufficient saline flush. A 2.7 F angioscope with a bending device was also developed (Fig. 2C). However, animal experiments revealed intimal damage induced by the wire by bending. Therefore, it was not used clinically. A 3.5 F and very flexible fiberscope with a guidewire slider at the distal-most tip was also developed (Fig. 2D).[1] This

angioscopy system greatly improved coaxiality. However, it was abandoned due to insufficient blood displacement. Many years later, a fiberscope with essentially the same structure was incorporated into a balloon-tipped inner guiding catheter in other institutions.

In these 4 angioscopy systems, the outer guiding catheter had no balloon at the distal tip. In order to occlude the proximal segment of coronary artery, balloon-tipped outer guiding catheters with or without side holes and with various configurations were developed (Fig. 3A-C).[2] Balloon-tipped inner guiding catheters with a steerable fiberscope and guidewire were also developed. In one system, the inner balloon catheter had one channel that allows introduction of the fiberscope, guidewire, and saline flush. Another inner guiding balloon catheter had 3 channels, one for the fiberscope, one for the guidewire, and the remaining one for saline flush or laser irradiation (Figs. 4A-C).

These inner balloon-guiding catheters enabled selective displacement of blood and greatly reduced flush volume. By pulling back the fiberscope, a considerable length of coronary artery could be observed during a single observation. Among them, the catheters shown in Fig. 4B and 4C are now frequently used in our catheterization laboratories.

Since manipulation of these 2 angioscopes are somewhat complicated, an angioscope with a fixed fiberscope on the inner guiding balloon catheter was also developed. This angioscope is now used for selected patients or for training.[3] To expand observation, the angioscope was separated into a fiberscope part and a balloon catheter part in which the former part can be advanced or pulled back over a guidewire for a considerable length during balloon inflation. This angioscope enabled successive observation

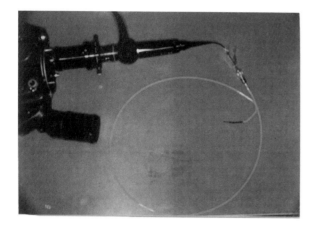

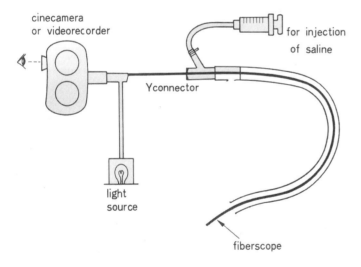

Fig. 1. An angioscopy system that was used for the first time for percutaneous observation of the changes in the proximal to the distal coronary segments.

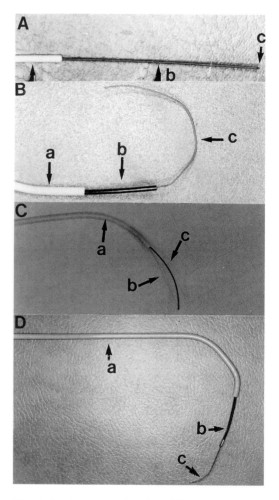

Fig. 2. Angioscopes developed in our laboratories. **A. a:** outer guiding catheter. **b:** inner guiding catheter. **c:** fiberscope. **B. a:** guiding catheter. **b:** fiberscope. **c:** guidewire. **C. a:** guiding catheter. **b:** fiberscope with metallic slider. **c:** guidewire.

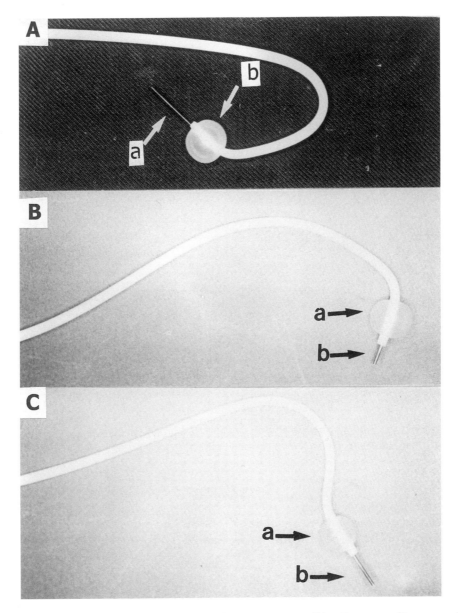

Fig. 3. Outer guiding balloon catheters developed in our laboratories. **A.** Judkins L type. **a:** fiberscope. **b:** guiding balloon catheter. **B.** Judkins R type. **a:** fiberscope. **b:** guiding balloon catheter. **C.** Amplatz L type. **a:** fiberscope. **b:** guiding balloon catheter.

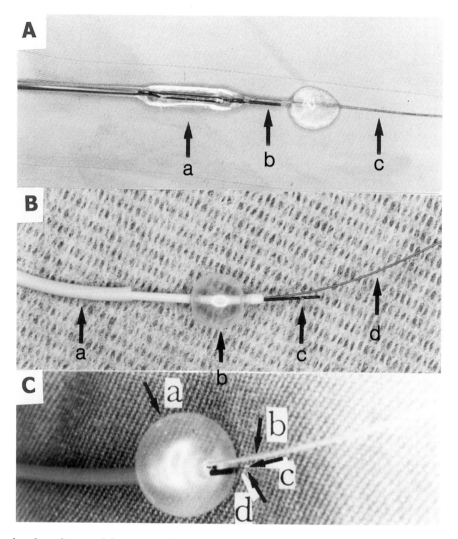

Fig. 4. Angioscopes developed in our laboratories. **A. a:** inner guiding catheter. **b:** fiberscope. **c:** guidewire. **B. a:** outer guiding catheter. **b:** inner guiding catheter. **c:** fiberscope. **d:** guidewire. **C. a:** inner guiding balloon catheter. **b:** guidewire. **c:** flush channel. **d:** fiberscope.

from the proximal to the distal segments. Dr. G. Abela showed me its prototype at Deaconess Hospital in Boston several years ago. This type of angioscope was much improved in our laboratories; the number of image fibers was increased to 4000 and then to 6000, and the fiberscope part became more flexible.

References

1. Uchida Y, Tomaru T, Sugimoto T: Observation of the coronary luminal changes induced by transluminal coronary angioplasty. Jpn Coll Angiol (Suppl):230, 1984 (abstract).

2. Uchida Y, Sugimoto T: Diagnosis of angina pectoris by percutaneous angioscopy. Clin Adult Dis 19:15–22, 1989.
3. Uchida Y: Atlas of Cardioangioscopy. Medical View Co, Tokyo, 1997.

Chapter 3

Coronary Angioscopy Systems and Their Manipulation:

Clinically Used Angioscopy Systems

An angioscopy system is composed of an angioscope, illumination source, CCD camera, image mixer, video recorder (tape or disc), and monitor. The angioscopy system we routinely use is shown in Fig. 1 and it is schematically shown in Fig. 2. By using a mixer, both angioscopic and fluoroscopic images are simultaneously recorded and monitored for identification of the location of the observed target (Fig. 3). The angioscope is composed of a fiberscope and guiding catheter with or without a balloon. At present, 3 types of angioscopes are frequently used for observation of coronary arteries in our laboratories.

Monorail Type Angioscope

Fig. 4 shows a commonly used monorail type angioscope. The angioscope is composed of the fiberscope part, the catheter part, and the fiberscope operation part (Fig. 5). The fiberscope contains 3000, 6000, or 8000 image guide silica fibers and 25 or 50 light guide (illumination) fibers. The fiberscope also has a guidewire slider at its distal-most tip, which allows a 0.014-inch guidewire to pass through (Fig. 6). By manipulating the fiberscope operation part, the fiberscope part can be advanced or pulled back over the wire for up to 6 cm (Fig. 4). The catheter part is 4.6 F in external diameter with an inflatable balloon at the distal-most tip, which is inflated with CO_2 to stop blood flow. The catheter part has a single lumen through which heparinized body temperature saline is infused manually or by a power injector to displace blood (Fig. 4).

This angioscope is introduced through an 8 F or 9 F outer guiding catheter, generally used for coronary interventions, into the coronary artery. Fig. 7 shows fluoroscopic images of the angioscope introduced into the coronary artery. Since there is a distance of about 1 cm from the balloon to the fiberscope tip, this angioscope is not feasible for observation of just the proximal segment including left main trunk (LMT). When this angioscope is used for observation of the proximal segment of the left anterior descending artery (LAD) or left circumflex artery (LCx), the LMT must be occluded with the balloon to obtain a sufficient visual field. This maneuver may cause global myocardial ischemia. In case of observation of LMT or the proximal segment of the right coronary artery (RCA), the balloon may locate in the outer guiding catheter, and therefore complete displacement of blood cannot be attained. Therefore, use of this angioscope is limited for observation of the middle to distal coronary segments in our laboratories[1] (Fig. 8).

Previously, we devised a 5 F balloon catheter with 3 lumens: 1 for the fiberscope, 1 for the guidewire, and the remaining 1 for the guidewire. Since both the fiberscope and the guidewire can be advanced or pulled back, manipulation of the guidewire under direct visualization can be performed (see Chapter 2, Fig. 4C).[2,3]

Fixed Type Angioscope

The catheter part is 4.6 F in diameter, has an inflatable balloon at the distal-most tip, and 2 lumens—one for the fiberscope, which contains 3000 or 6000 silica fibers and the other for 0.014 guidewire and saline flush. Since the fiberscope is fixed on the catheter, it can be manipulated more easily than the

11

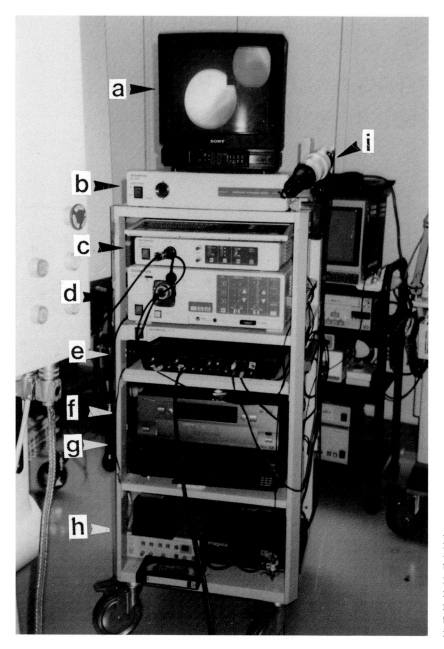

Fig. 1. Angioscopy system used in our laboratory. **a:** monitor. **b:** intracardiac ultrasound system (ICUS). **c:** CCD camera for angioscopy and cardioscopy. **d:** illumination source. **e:** image mixer. **f:** DVD recorder. **h:** fluorescence image controller. **i:** ICCD camera for fluorescence image angioscopy and cardioscopy.

monorail type angioscope (Fig. 9). This type of angioscope is also used for observation of the middle to distal coronary segments, and is relatively feasible for observation of the proximal segments (Fig. 8). If the angioscope is pulled back without balloon inflation during saline infusion, the proximal segments of LAD, LCx, and RCA can be observed.[3]

In this type, observation during one balloon inflation is limited to a confined portion because the angioscope cannot be moved during balloon inflation. If the angioscope is moved during balloon inflation, endothelial denudation may be induced.

Bare Fiberscope With Outer Guiding Catheter With or Without Balloon

The angioscope is composed of a 5 F fiberscope with 4000 or 6000 image fibers or 2.6 F fiberscope with 3000 or 4000 image fibers and guiding catheter. A larger fiberscope is more suitable for bull's eye observation since coaxiality can more easily be obtained with a larger fiberscope. This angioscope is simple and was first used in our laboratory,[4] and is very useful for observation of the proximal coronary segments including LMT and also for observation of cardiac

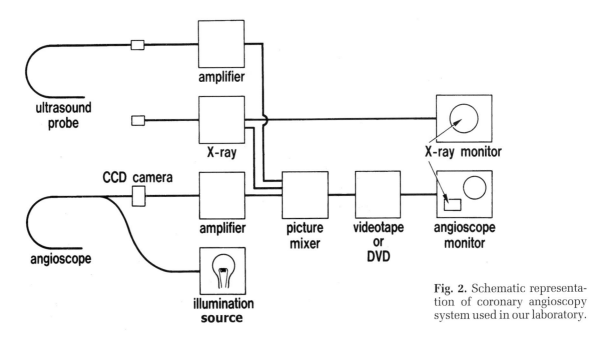

Fig. 2. Schematic representation of coronary angioscopy system used in our laboratory.

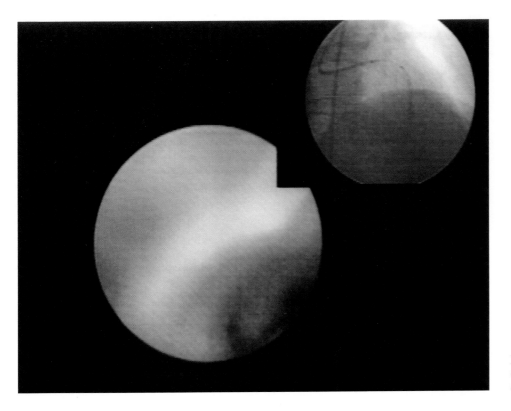

Fig. 3. Simultaneously recorded angioscopic and x-ray images using a mixer.

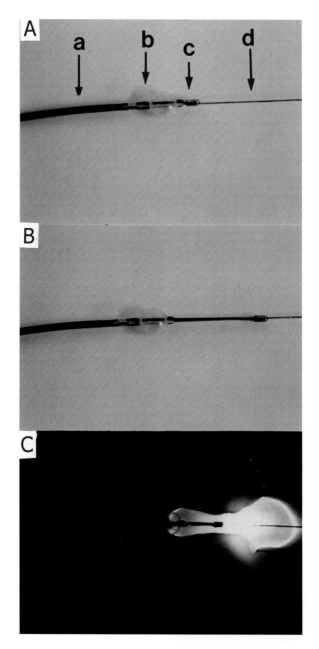

Fig. 4. Monorail type angioscope. **A:** fiberscope part pulled back. **a:** catheter part. **b:** balloon. **c:** fiberscope part. **d:** guidewire. **B:** fiberscope part advanced. **C:** saline flush.

chambers and great vessels (Fig. 8, Chapter 20). Since a larger amount of saline is required for blood displacement, use of a power injector is recommended.

Fluorescence Image Angioscopy Systems

Various substances composing the vascular wall exhibit autofluorescence when excited by corresponding rays with specific lengths. Also, they can be labeled with fluorescent dyes. Therefore, there is a possibility that individual cells or substances composing the nonatherosclerotic and atherosclerotic plaques can be discriminated by fluorescence images or by spectral analysis. In addition, by targeting autofluorescence or labeled fluorescence, the targeted cells or substances can be vaporized by laser irradiation.

Fig. 10 shows a fluorescence image angioscopy system that we devised for intravascular use. The fluorescence angioscope is essentially the same as that of the monorail type (Fig. 5).

This angioscope is connected to an illumination source (Xe-Hg lamp) and ICCD camera. By changing excitation filters incorporated in the illumination source, excitation rays can be changed from 320 to 750 nm. Also, by changing cut filters, fluorescence images from 370 to 880 nm can be obtained. When filters for fluorescence are not used, usual visual light images can be obtained.[5]

Dye Image Angioscopy

Magnification of conventional angioscopes for coronary use is up to ×30 and the number of image fibers is limited due to the thin external diameter. Therefore, discrimination of small lesions are beyond them. However, with the aid of dyes that selectively stain a given cell, tissue, or substance, small lesions can be discriminated even by conventional angioscopes.

During a search for dyes specifically to stain damaged endothelial cells, we found that Evans blue, which was used for assessment of cardiac output in patients, selectively stains damaged endothelial cells and fibrin in vivo.[6]

After routine angioscopy, 1 mL of 2% or 5% Evans blue solution is injected into the coronary artery through the flush lumen during balloon inflation; after 5 seconds, saline is flushed for observation. By this maneuver, damaged endothelial cells and fibrin are stained in blue. Tripan blue, which is used for treatment of *Tripanozoma* infection, can also be used for the same purpose.

Vascular endothelial cells are easily damaged by mechanical interventions. Even a very floppy and soft-tipped guidewire used for coronary interventions can damage the endothelial cells.[7] Therefore, in case of observation of damaged endothelial cells, the guidewire should not be advanced prior to advancement of the angioscope. However, introduction of an angioscope without a guidewire is dangerous because once obstruction by an angioscope occurs, immediate rescue recanalization is often difficult. Therefore, use of a guidewire is essential. To achieve these 2 conflicting purposes, use of a Magnum wire,

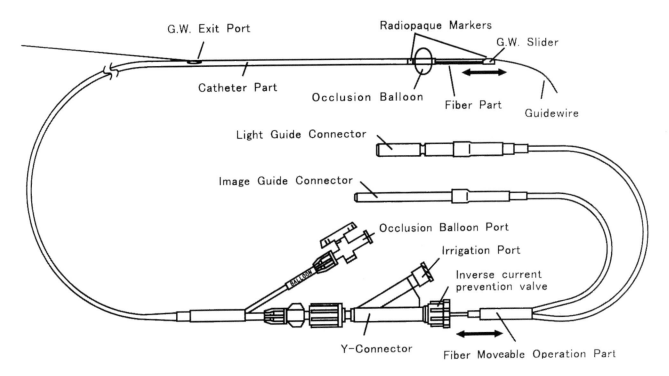

Fig. 5. Schematic representation of the monorail type angioscope. G.W.: guidewire.

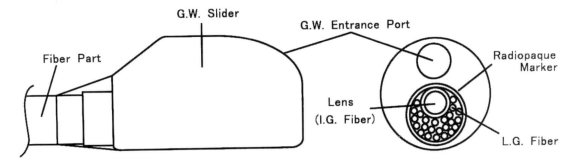

Fig. 6. Schematic representation of the distal-most tip of the fiberscope part. I.G.: image guide. L.G.: light guide.

which has a small ball at the distal-most tip, is recommended because a ball tip prevents detachment of the wire itself from the angioscope. A Magnum wire is introduced into the guidewire slider of the angioscope so as to locate its ball tip close to the slider, the angioscope is advanced to a segment proximal to the target lesion, the balloon is inflated and Evans blue is injected, and the fiberscope part is advanced, now guided by the wire during saline flush for observation of endothelial damages. When accidental obstruction is induced, the wire can immediately be advanced to secure the true lumen for recanalization.

Identification of Location of the Target Lesion

Use of a guidewire with markers by 0.5- or 1-cm increments and angiograms obtained during angioscopy are used for identification of the location of the angioscope tip and the target lesion. However, shorter axis location of the target lesion is sometimes difficult. When the target lesion is located close to a side branch, identification of the location of the target lesion is easy.

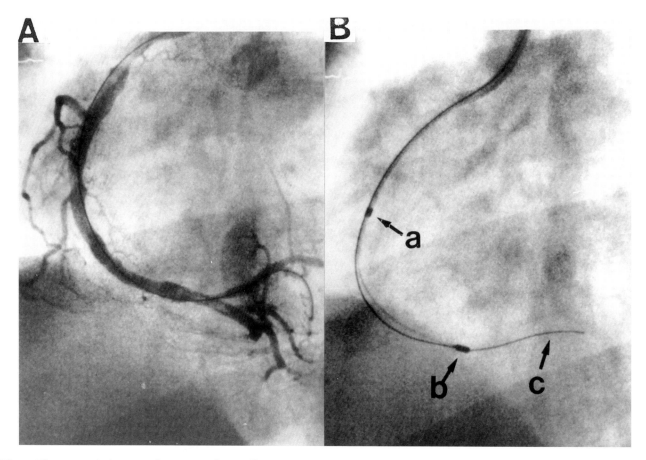

Fig. 7. Fluoroscopic images of a monorail type fiberscope that was introduced into the RCA. **A:** coronary angiogram. **B:** angioscope. **a:** catheter part. **b:** fiberscope part. **c:** guidewire.

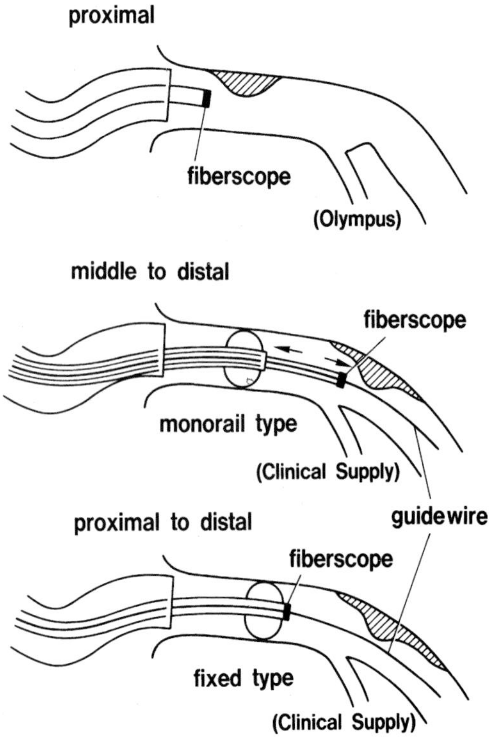

Fig. 8. Schematic representation of manipulation of the 3 different angioscopes. From top: bare fiberscope, monorail type angioscope, and fixed type angioscope.

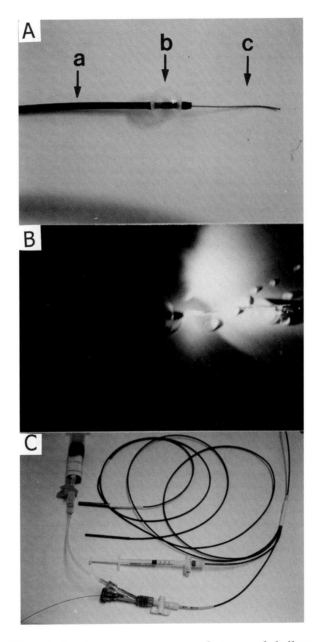

Fig. 9. A: fixed type angioscope. **a:** catheter part. **b:** balloon. **c:** guidewire. **B:** during saline flush. **C:** proximal end of angioscope.

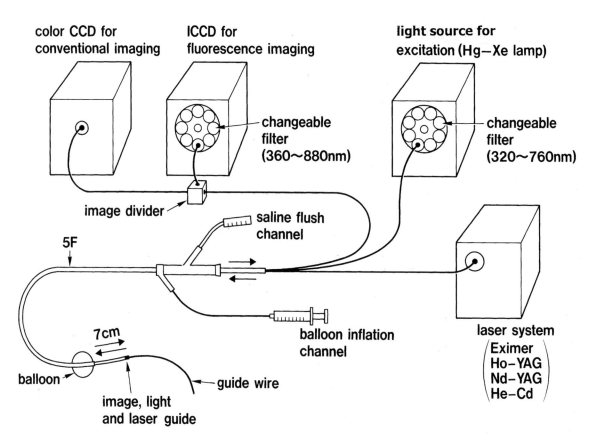

Fig. 10. Schematic representation of fluorescence image angioscopy system.

Calibration

Fig. 11 shows a section paper observed by a conventional angioscope. The magnification rate at the center of the visual field is larger than those of peripheral portions. Also, regional differences in magnification are exaggerated when the distance between the angioscope tip and the target becomes smaller. In addition, since the lens is handmade, the magnification rate may differ from lens to lens. Therefore, quantitative measurement of target size is very difficult. Nevertheless, approximate size of the target can be obtained by comparing the diameter of the guidewire located on the target and the target itself. In the near future, quantitative analyzers may be used.

Color Correction

The CCD amplifier contains color bars and also an automatic white balancer. It is convenient to use gauze as a white target. By pushing the white bal-

ancer during targeting the gauze at a distance of 5 mm, good white balance can be obtained.

When illumination output, namely light guide output, is excessive, any target becomes white due to halation, and adjustment of light guide output by using a graded output controller is necessary. Brightness of the target lesion is influenced by the diameter of the coronary segment, surrounding tissues, and the target itself.

Since discrimination of color is rather subjective, quantitative colorimetric analyzers should be used in the future.[8]

Sterilization

All angioscopes except bare fiberscopes are for single use and are sterilized with EGO and packed in a box, similar to intravascular ultrasound (IVUS) catheters. Since bare fiberscopes can be used repeatedly, they are sterilized with EGO before use, or stored in 4% glutaraldehyde solution for 4 hours for

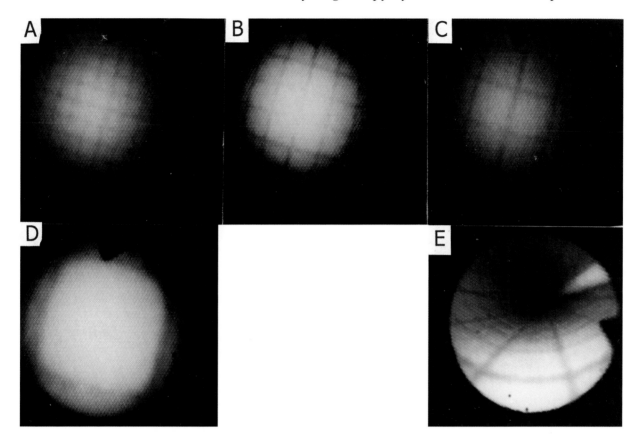

Fig. 11. Angioscopic images of section papers, showing nonuniform magnification of the target. From **A** to **D**: 10, 5, 3, 1 mm from the target. **E**: interior of a tube made of a section paper.

sterilization.[3] Bare fiberscopes should not be reused after their use in patients with infectious diseases.

Premedication

Premedication is essentially the same as that for coronary interventions such as plain old balloon [coronary] angioplasty (POBA) and stenting. Before transferring to the catheterization laboratory, the patients are given oral diazepam. Immediately after introduction of the sheath into the femoral or radial artery, heparin (5000 IU) is injected intravenously. Intravenous injection of lidocaine 50 mg and intracoronary injection of nitroglycerin 200 µg are also performed just before coronary angioscopy. Larger doses of heparin and lidocaine may be necessary for certain patients, due to larger bodyweight.

Procedures

After diagnostic coronary angiography with 5 F or 6 F catheters, the sheath in the right femoral artery is replaced by an 8 F. Then, an 8 F guiding catheter for coronary interventions is introduced through the sheath into the aortic root so as to locate its tip in the ostium of the coronary artery. Then, one of the angioscopes shown in Figs. 4 and 9 is introduced through the guiding catheter into the coronary artery. An angioscope appropriate for observation of the given plaque is selected and angioscopy is performed as described in the following sections.

Selection of Guiding Catheters

After confirmation of the target plaque for observation, the 6 F sheath is replaced by a 8 F sheath, through which an 8 F guiding catheter for PTCA use is introduced into the aortic root so as to locate its distal tip in the coronary ostium. In general, an Amplatz catheter is more suitable for the left coronary artery. In the right coronary artery, the suitable catheter is dependent on its branching angle to the aorta. A Judkins catheter is suitable for horizontal or downward branching and an Amplatz catheter for upright branching. A guiding catheter with side holes is recommended when the ostium is narrow.

Angioscopy of Middle to Distal Coronary Segments

The first choice for middle to distal segments is a monorail type angioscope (Fig. 4). A 0.014 guidewire is advanced across the plaque. Then, the angioscope is advanced carefully over the guidewire so as to locate the tip of the fiberscope part just proximal to the target plaque, and the balloon is located in the proximal segment and not in the LMT (in the case of left coronary artery). Use of a guidewire with markers at every 1 cm is recommended for confirmation of the location of the plaque and the fiberscope tip. A fiberscope tip is easily identified by its metallic slider and the balloon by a marker (Fig. 7). When the angioscope is properly located, the balloon is inflated manually. Usually, 0.5 mL of carbon dioxide is enough for complete occlusion. Then, heparinized and warmed saline is infused. Manual infusion of saline using a plastic syringe containing 20 mL of saline is recommended because infusion speed can be controlled during observation and excessive infusion can be prevented. Use of a power injector may be beneficial when there are fewer than 3 operators. However, special care should be taken not to infuse saline when the fiberscope part is at the completely pulled-back position. In this situation, an excessive increase of pressure within the catheter part occurs and, accordingly, shaft perforation may occur.

When the blood is completely displaced with saline, clear visualization of the coronary interior will be obtained. One to 2 seconds are required for complete blood displacement. Then, the fiberscope part is slowly advanced over the wire, confirming the wall changes successively. Observation of the coronary luminal surface by advancing the fiberscope part resembles observation of the tunnel wall from a running train. We usually stop advancement of the fiberscope tip when the target plaque becomes very close. When the narrowing is moderate to mild, we advance it across the plaque more distally. After observation by advancing the fiberscope part, the balloon is deflated and saline infusion is stopped to prevent excessive ischemia and serious arrhythmias.

When the electrocardiogram returns to the control state, the balloon is again inflated and saline is infused to observe the same target by pulling back the fiberscope part. When the coronary segment to be observed is tortuous or angled, the fiberscope part is advanced under fluoroscopic guidance and observation is performed by pulling back the fiberscope part for prevention of the coronary wall damage by advancing. When the fiberscope part cannot be advanced, rotation of the catheter part or advancement with guidewire may be helpful. When halation of the target plaque occurs, reduction in illumination output is required for evaluation of color of the target.

Marked elongation of the QT interval and giant negative T always appear during saline infusion. However, they disappear promptly on deflation of the balloon. Infusion of less than 20 mL and balloon occlusion time less than 30 seconds for single observation are safe.

Angioscopy of Proximal Coronary Segments Including LMT

The first choice for observation of the LMT and the proximal segment of the right coronary artery is an 8 F outer guiding catheter with side holes. The catheter is introduced into the segment so as to locate the tip in the artery close to the ostium. Then, a bare fiberscope is introduced through the catheter into the artery. We prefer a 5 F fiberscope to obtain coaxiality. Use of a guidewire is unnecessary. Then, saline is infused by a power injector at a rate of 3–4 mL/sec for 4–5 sec. During saline infusion, the fiberscope is advanced or pulled back for observation. The second choice is a monorail type angioscope. The fiberscope part is located in the segment and the catheter part is located in the outer guiding catheter. Saline is infused through the outer guiding catheter without balloon inflation.

Angioscopy of a Bypass Graft

The procedure for angioscopy of a bypass graft is quite similar to that of the native coronary artery. Successive observation from the graft ostium to the junction of the native artery can be performed.

Angioscopy During Coronary Interventions

Angioscopy of the coronary lesions before and after intervention are generally performed for selection of therapeutic modalities and for evaluation of interventions. The techniques to exchange the angioscope to therapeutic catheters and vice versa are easy.

Dye Image Angioscopy

Evans blue dye is the sole dye used. The safety and usefulness of Evans blue dye has been proven and it is used for identification of endothelial cell damage and fibrin. Endothelial cells are very fragile and are easily damaged even by a gentle mechanical stimulus; therefore, neither the angioscope nor the guidewire tip should touch the target before observation. To attain this purpose and to secure prompt recanalization once obstruction accidentally occurs during angioscope manipulation, we usually use a ball-tipped Magnum guidewire. The wire is introduced into the metallic guidewire slider of the monorail type angioscope so as to locate the ball tip at the outlet of the slider. The ball prevents the wire from dropping off. The angioscope is advanced just proximal to the target. Then, the balloon is inflated and 1 mL of 2% or 5% Evans blue solution is injected through the flush channel of the angioscope. After 5 seconds, the balloon is deflated.

Thirty seconds later, the balloon is inflated and observation is repeated. By this maneuver, endothelial cells damaged by other causes and fibrin can be observed in blue. In the future, differential vital staining of various cells and substances may be established.

Fluorescent Image Angioscopy

After routine observation, the CCD camera is changed to an ICCD camera and excitation filters and cut filters are changed as wanted while the angioscope is placed at the same position. By infusing saline, an autofluorescent image can be obtained.

Local administration of fluorescent dye is another choice for observation of specific substances. Since affinity to platelets and fibrin is very strong, we inject 0.5 mL of 1% FITC solution into the coronary artery through the outer guiding catheter for identification of platelets and fibrin. In dogs, eosin also stains platelets in purple when administered with Evans blue, and its fluorescence can also be detected. However, its clinical safety is unknown. Hematoporphyrin derivative (porfimer sodium) is absorbed into the atheroma and radiates red fluorescence when excited with a 630-nm ray.[9]

Combined Use of Angioscopy and Intravascular Ultrasound

By changing the angioscope to an IVUS catheter, the surface and wall morphology of the same plaque can be examined.

Complications

During saline infusion, giant negative T, extreme elongation of the QT segment, and elevation or depression of the ST segment of the electrocardiogram always occur (Fig.12). When elongation of the QT segment and T inversion appear, we immediately deflate the balloon and stop saline infusion. On deflation of the balloon and cessation of saline infusion, they promptly disappear. According to our experience, appearance of advanced ventricular arrhythmia is very rare when the patients are premedicated with lidocaine. Table 1 shows serious complications experienced in our laboratories in the past 20 years.

Endothelial cells become very weak when exposed to mechanical stimuli, and even a very floppy guidewire for coronary intervention causes endothelial damage. Fig.13 shows endothelial damages induced by a 0.014 guidewire for PTCA use and those induced by inflation of an angioscope balloon.[7]

What Should and Should Not Be Done

1. Since the conventional angioscopes are rather stiff, a segment with an angle of 90° or more should not be passed through by the angioscope to avoid coronary artery dissection or fracture of the fiberscope part.

2. Abrupt halation of the entire visual field during manipulation indicates a touch of the lens to the luminal surface. In this case, the fiberscope part should be pulled back to avoid damage to the vascular wall.

3. When yellow and glittering substances occupy the entire visual field, especially in the case of a bare fiberscope, the fiberscope tip is within the vascular wall. Therefore, the fiberscope should not be advanced farther to avoid perforation and should immediately be pulled back. In this case, angiography should be performed to confirm whether perforation or vascular wall damage has occurred.

4. When thrombus is observed on the guidewire, the wire and angioscope should be withdrawn. Removal of the guidewire alone may induce detachment of the thrombus and may cause distal embolization (Fig. 14).

5. Small air bubbles are often observed during saline infusion. They are usually not harmful. However, when a bubble occupies the entire visual field as shown in Fig. 14, it indicates either gas embolism with

accidental air injection, or CO_2 due to balloon rupture. In this case, the angioscope should be withdrawn and the infusion route and the balloon should be checked.

6. When giant negative T and extreme elongation of the QT segment of the electrocardiogram appear, the balloon should be immediately deflated and saline infusion should be stopped.

7. In case of LMT observation, observation should be stopped when bradycardia or a fall in systemic blood pressure occur.

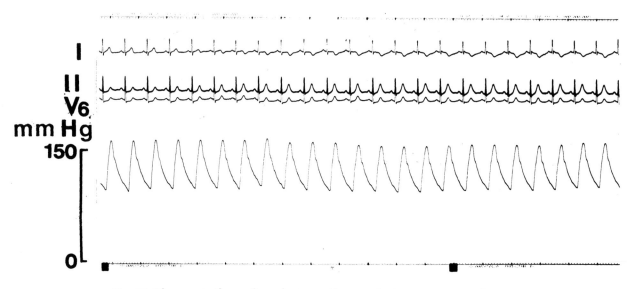

Fig. 12. Changes in the surface electrocardiogram during coronary angioscopy.

Table 1
Complications of Percutaneous Coronary Angioscopy

	Chest Pain Syndromes	SA	UA	AMI	Chronic Stage of AMI	Kawasaki Disease	Total
	n = 42	380	64	81	73	9	649
Dissection		3			2		5
Acute closure		1	1		1*		3
AMI		2				1	3
VT,VF							
Death					1**		1
Total	0	6(1.6%)	1(1.6%)		4(5.4%)	1(11.1%)	12(1.9%)

SA: stable angina pectoris. UA: unstable angina pectoris. AMI: acute myocardial infarction. VT: ventricular tachycardia. VF: ventricular fibrillation. *: acute closure of POBA site on repeated angioscopy 6 months later.
**: same patient as that labeled with *: Death due to cardiac tamponade after surgery.

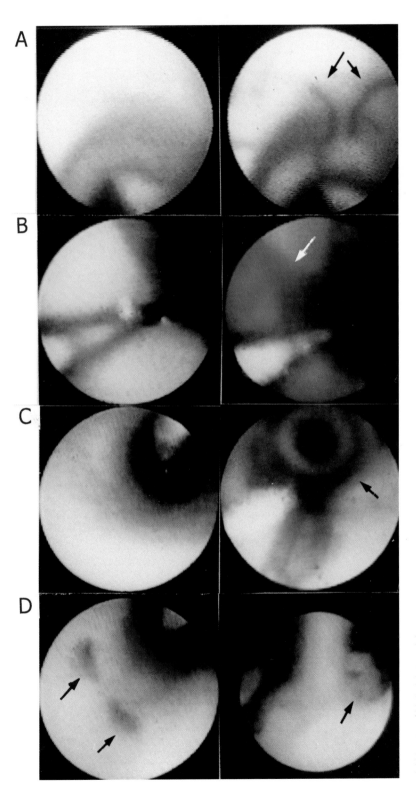

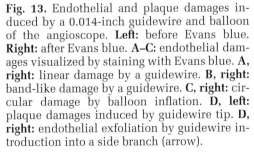

Fig. 13. Endothelial and plaque damages induced by a 0.014-inch guidewire and balloon of the angioscope. **Left:** before Evans blue. **Right:** after Evans blue. **A–C:** endothelial damages visualized by staining with Evans blue. **A, right:** linear damage by a guidewire. **B, right:** band-like damage by a guidewire. **C, right:** circular damage by balloon inflation. **D, left:** plaque damages induced by guidewire tip. **D, right:** endothelial exfoliation by guidewire introduction into a side branch (arrow).

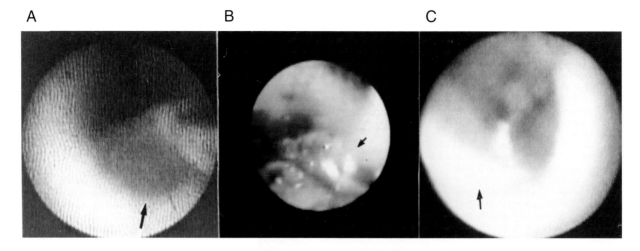

Fig. 14. A: thrombus formation on the guidewire. **B:** small and multiple bubbles. **C:** a large bubble occupying the lumen.

References

1. Fujimori Y, Uchida Y: Intracoronary imaging. In: Cardiovascular Catheterization. Nakayama Publishing Co., Tokyo, 1998, pp 499–503.
2. Uchida Y, Fujimori Y, Hirose J, et al: Percutaneous coronary angioscopy. Jpn Heart J 33:271–294, 1992.
3. Uchida Y: Cardioangioscopy. Medical View Co., Tokyo, 1995, pp 20–30.
4. Uchida Y, Tomaru T, Nakamura F, et al: Percutaneous coronary angioscopy in patients with ischemic heart disease. Am Heart J 114:216–1222, 1987.
5. Uchida Y: Fluorescence image coronary angioscopy. Jpn Circulat J 75(Suppl): 1999.
6. Uchida Y, Nakamura F, Morita T: Observation of atherosclerotic lesions by intravascular microscope in patients with arteriosclerosis obliterans. Am Heart J 130:1114–1119, 1995.
7. Terasawa K, Fujimori Y, Morio H, et al: Evaluation of coronary endothelial cell damages caused by PTCA guidewires by in vivo dye staining angioscopy. J Jpn Coll Angiol 40:159–164, 2000.
8. Lehmann KG, van Suylen RJ, Stibbe J, et al: Composition of human thrombus assessed by quantitative colorimetric analysis. Circulation 96: 3030–3041, 1997.
9. Amemiya T, Nakajima H, Katoh T, et al: Photodynamic therapy using YAG-OPO laser and porfimer sodium, and comparison with using Argon-dye laser. Jpn Circulat J 63: 288–295, 1999.

Chapter 4

Histological Aspects of Evolution and Progression of Atherosclerotic Coronary Plaques

Histological classification, evolution, and progression of a therosclerotic lesions were recommended by the American Heart Association Council on Arteriosclerosis (Table 1; Fig. 1).[1] According to the recommendation, the initial (type I) lesion contains enough atherogenic lipoprotein to elicit an increase in macrophages and formation of scattered foam cells. Type II lesions consist primarily of layers of macrophage foam cells and lipid-laden smooth muscle cells and include lesions grossly designated as fatty streaks. Type III is the intermediate stage between type II and type IV; these lesions contain scattered collections of extracellular lipid droplets. In type IV lesions (atheroma), a dense accumulation of extracellular lipid occupies an extensive but well-defined region of intima that is called lipid core or lipid pool, and complications such as defects of lesion surface or thrombosis are not present, and the tissue layer between the lipid core and endothelial surface is still largely the intima that preceded lesion development.

The potential clinical significance of this type is vulnerability to disruption due to minimal collagen between the lipid core and the endothelium.[2,3] Whether this type is identical to the glistening yellow plaque of our angioscopic classification remains to be clarified (see Chapter 5). Type V lesions are defined as lesions in which prominent new fibrous connective tissue has formed. When new fibrous tissue is formed in type IV lesions, this is called type Va (fibroatheroma). A type V lesion in which the lipid core

and other parts are calcified is referred to as type Vb. A type V lesion in which a lipid core is absent is referred to as type Vc. Type VI or V lesions associated with disruptions of the surface, hematoma, hemorrhage, and or thrombosis are classified as type VI (complicated or complex). This type is further subdivided into type VIa (disruption), type VIb (hematoma or hemorrhage), and type VIc (thrombosis). Since time course changes in the same atherosclerotic lesions, especially coronary lesions, have never been examined histologically, there is a possibility that a certain group of lesions may take pathways other than the normal pathways.

Clinically, atherosclerotic lesions are called "plaques," and. therefore, we use this term instead of "lesions." Angioscopically, we call atherosclerotic lesions "plaque" when their prominence is obvious. Also, we call the lesions "plaques" by IVUS when the intima is more than 0.25 mm in thickness, irrespective of their angiographic prominence into the lumen. Therefore, there are discrepancies in definition among angioscopy, IVUS and angiography, and histology.

As to lipid pool or core, we call them the "lipid pool," because there are lipid depositions that are not positioned at the center of the plaque.

Also, the plaques without visible surface disruption, hematoma, hemorrhage, and thrombosis by conventional angioscopy or IVUS are referred to as regular (uncomplicated) plaques, and those with visible surface disruption are referred to as complex (complicated) plaques.

Table 1
Terms Used to Designate Different Types of Human Atherosclerotic Lesions in Pathology

Terms for Atherosclerotic Lesions in Histological Classification	Other Terms for the Same Lesions Based on Appearance With the Unaided Eyes
Type I lesion initial lesion	
Type IIa lesion progression prone	fatty dot or streak, early lesion
Type IIb lesion progression resistant	
Type III lesion intermediate lesion (preatheroma)	
Type IV lesion atheroma lesion	atheromatous plaque, fibrolipid plaque, fibrous plaque, plaque
Type Va lesion fibroatheroma	
Vb calcific lesion (type VII lesion)	calcified plaque,
Vc fibrotic lesion (type VIII lesion)	fibrotic plaque
Type VI lesion lesions with surface defect, and/or hematoma hemorrhage, and/or thrombotic deposit	complicated lesion, complicated plaque

Used with permission from ref. 1.

Nomenclature and main histology	Sequences in progression	Main growth mechanism	Earliest onset	Clinical corre-lation
Type I (initial) lesion isolated macrophage foam cells	I	growth mainly by lipid accumu-lation	from first decade	clinically silent
Type II (fatty streak) lesion mainly intracellular lipid accumulation	II			
Type III (intermediate) lesion Type II changes & small extracellular lipid pools	III		from third decade	
Type IV (atheroma) lesion Type II changes & core of extracellular lipid	IV			
Type V (fibroatheroma) lesion lipid core & fibrotic layer, or multiple lipid cores & fibrotic layers, or mainly calcific, or mainly fibrotic	V	accelerated smooth muscle and collagen increase	from fourth decade	clinically silent or overt
Type VI (complicated) lesion surface defect, hematoma-hemorrhage, thrombus	VI	thrombosis, hematoma		

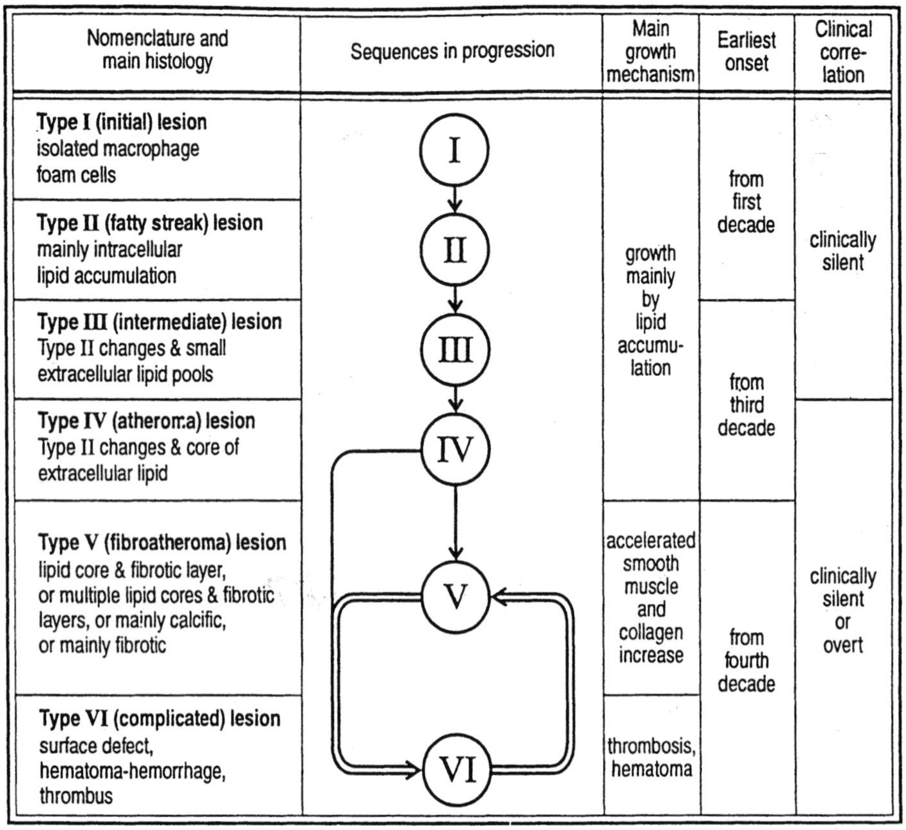

Fig. 1. Classification and pathways in evolution and progression of human atherosclerotic lesions. Used with permission from ref. 1.

References

1. Stary HC, Chandler AB, Dinsmore RE, et al: A definition of advanced types of atherosclerotic lesions and a histological classification of atherosclerosis: A Report from the Committee on Vascular Lesions of the Council on Arteriosclerosis, American Heart Association. Circulation 92: 1355–1374, 1995.

2. Constantinides P: Plaque fissuring in human coronary thrombosis. J Atheroscler Res 6:1–17, 1966.

3. Falk E: Morphologic features of unstable atherothrombotic plaques underlying acute coronary syndromes. Am J Cardiol 63:114E-120E, 1989.

Chapter 5

Histological Basis for Interpretation of Angioscopic and Ultrasonographic (IVUS) Images of Atherosclerotic Coronary Plaques

Relationships Among Angioscopic, Intravascular Ultrasonographic (IVUS) Images and Histological Changes of Coronary Plaques

Considerable knowledge has been accumulated on the intravascular ultrasonographic images of coronary plaques and their correlations to histological changes; however, there are no systematic studies on the relationships between angioscopic images and histological changes.

In clinical situations, coronary plaques are angioscopically classified into regular (nondisrupted) and complex (disrupted) plaques.[1] Regular (nondisrupted) coronary atherosclerotic plaques are classified by color as white (W), light yellow (LY), yellow (Y), brown (B), and glistening yellow plaques (GY). Those brown in color are usually included in yellow.[2] However, pathological characteristics of these different categories of plaques are not well determined. Therefore, we examined the relationships between angioscopic images, especially surface color, and histological changes of the removed human coronary arteries to determine what category of plaques is histologically vulnerable.

We found that lipids and calcium are simultaneously stained with oil red O followed by hematoxylin, respectively, into red and dark purple. Therefore, instead of von Kossa's method, which is generally used for calcium staining,[3] we used this method for identification of their deposition sites and relationships between them in the same plaques. Collagen and elastic fibers were stained by Ag and EVG stain, respectively. Since macrophages act to destabilize the atherosclerotic plaques, ceroids, intermediate metabolites of lipids produced by macrophages, were stained by Tiel-Nielzen stain.[4] The plaque stain results were histologically classified into nonlipid pool and lipid pool types.

Fig. 1 shows a representative regular white plaque without a lipid pool inside. By IVUS, the plaque shows a concentric stenosis and is highly echoic (hard). Histologically, the plaque is almost devoid of lipids and ceroids, and is rich and dense in normal collagen and elastic fibers. Since collagen fibers are believed to protect the plaque from disruption, this finding indicates that this plaque is stable.

Fig. 2 shows a white plaque with a lipid pool inside. The fibrous cap covering the pool is thick and rich in collagen fibers, and except those close to the lipid pool, collagen fibers are normal. Lipid and calcium deposition is limited to the margin of the lipid pool and it is not found in the superficial layers of the fibrous cap. These histological changes indicate that this plaque is stable. Fig. 3 shows a white plaque protruding into the lumen. By IVUS, a thick superficial calcium layer is observed. Histologically, a large lipid pool is wrapped by a thick calcium armor. The armor seems to be located just beneath the endothelium. Although devoid of normal collagen fibers, the plaque seems relatively stable because a tight calcium armor may protect the lipid pool from disruption.

Fig. 4 shows a light yellow plaque without a lipid pool. It is isoechoic by IVUS. Lipids are deposited diffusely in deeper layers. Collagen fibers are densely distributed and calcium and ceroids are not observable in the superficial layers. This plaque is considered stable.

Fig. 5 shows a nonglistening yellow plaque with-

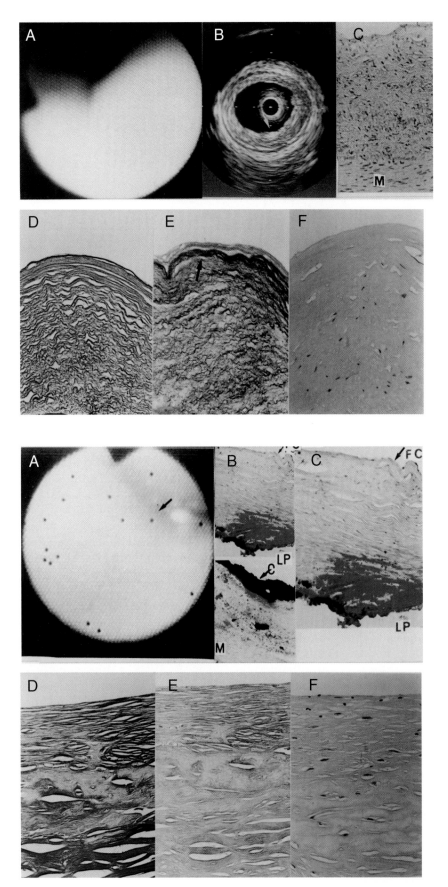

Fig. 1. A: angioscopy. White plaque without lipid pool. B: IVUS. Hard plaque. C: oil red O and hematoxylin stain. ×100. No lipid deposition. No lipid pool. M: media; D: Ag stain. Rich in collagen fibers (purplish red). E: EVG stain. Internal elastic lamina (arrow) and elastic fibers (dark blue). F: Tiel-Nielzen staining. No ceroids. ×400.

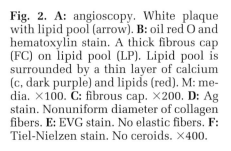

Fig. 2. A: angioscopy. White plaque with lipid pool (arrow). B: oil red O and hematoxylin stain. A thick fibrous cap (FC) on lipid pool (LP). Lipid pool is surrounded by a thin layer of calcium (c, dark purple) and lipids (red). M: media. ×100. C: fibrous cap. ×200. D: Ag stain. Nonuniform diameter of collagen fibers. E: EVG stain. No elastic fibers. F: Tiel-Nielzen stain. No ceroids. ×400.

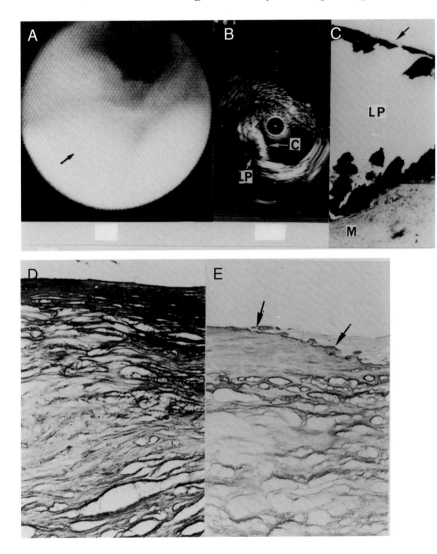

Fig. 3. A: angioscopy. White plaque (arrow). **B:** IVUS. A thick superficial calcium layer (c) with shadow behind. **C:** oil red O and hematoxylin stain. Calcium deposition just beneath the endothelium (arrow) with lipid pool (LP) that corresponds to that in B. The thick calcium layer on the media (M) observed histologically in C was hidden by the shadow of superficial calcium layer in B. ×100. **D:** Ag stain after decalcification. All collagen fibers are degenerated. **E:** Tiel-Nielzen stain after decalcification. No ceroids. Diffuse purplish area (arrows) indicates calcium-deposited portion. ×400.

out a lipid pool. By IVUS, it is a low echoic plaque. Lipids are deposited diffusely from the superficial to the deep layers; however, calcium and ceroids are not found. The collagen fibers are densely distributed. However, the diameter of the fibers is irregular and those superficially located are degenerated. This plaque is considered rather fragile when compared to white plaques.

Fig. 6 shows a glistening yellow plaque. The plaque is protruding like a yellow water droplet into the lumen and glistens, reflecting illumination.

By IVUS, an echolucent space beneath a layer with nonuniform echogenicity is observed. Histologically, a lipid pool is surrounded by a calcium armor that cannot be identified by IVUS. The fibrous cap covering the armor is deposited with lipids and fine calcium particles. Collagen fibers are scarce and degenerated or atrophied, and ceroids are densely deposited. This plaque is considered vulnerable. The

cap with relatively higher echogenicity than the lipid pool despite loss of collagen fibers may be due to disseminated deposition of fine calcium crystals.

Fig. 7 shows a glistening yellow plaque that protruded into the lumen. The surface was somewhat turbid and a small delle is observed. By IVUS, the plaque is observed to be low echoic and a high echoic mass without shadow is located laterally. Histologically, the fibrous cap is extremely thin and abundant with lipids, fine calcium particles, and ceroids. Collagen fibers are few in number and they are atrophic, indicating that this plaque is extremely vulnerable. A small pore in the cap that corresponds to the delle in the angioscopic image and bleeding inside indicates ongoing disruption.

Fig. 8 also shows a glistening yellow plaque not protruding into the lumen. By IVUS, the plaque is isoechoic. The plaque is devoid of a lipid pool inside, and lipid deposition is restricted to the superficial

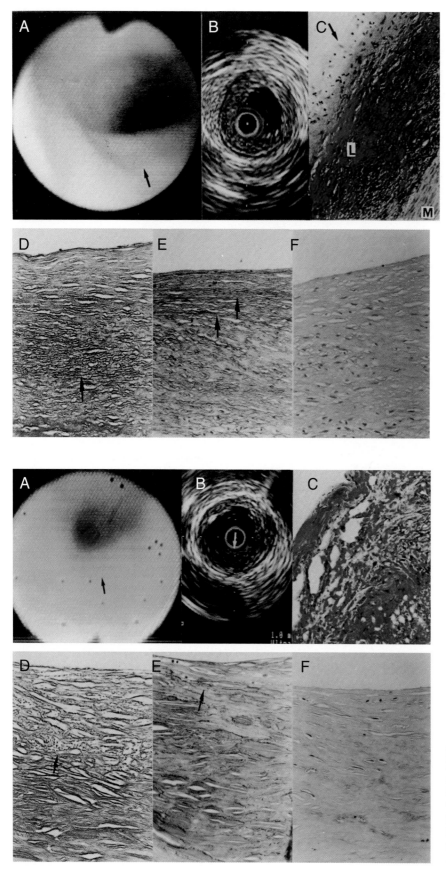

Fig. 4. A: angioscopy. Light yellow plaque (arrow). **B:** IVUS. Rather high echoic concentric plaque. **C:** oil red O and hematoxylin stain. Diffuse lipid deposition (L) except superficial layer without a lipid pool. The lipid may have been seen through a thin lipid-absent superficial layer (arrow). ×100. **M:** media. **D:** Ag stain. Atrophic collagen fibers in the middle layer (arrow). **E:** EVG stain. Elastic fibers present (arrows). ×400. **F:** Tiel-Nielzen stain. No ceroids. ×400.

Fig. 5. A: angioscopy. Nonglistening yellow plaque (arrow). **B:** IVUS. Soft concentric plaque. **C:** oil red O and hematoxylin stain. Diffuse lipid deposition without a lipid pool. ×100. **D:** Ag stain. Disrupted collagen fibers (arrow). **E:** EVG stain. Disrupted elastic fibers (arrow). **F:** Tiel-Nielzen stain. No ceroids. ×400.

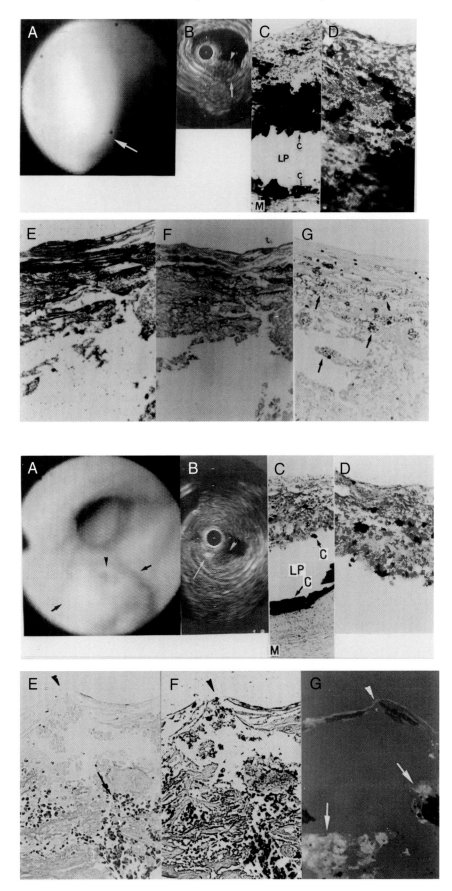

Fig. 6. A: angioscopy. Glistening yellow plaque. **B:** IVUS. A low echoic space (arrow) covered with a relatively high echoic fibrous cap (arrowhead). **C:** oil red O and hematoxylin stain. A loose fibrous cap deposited with lipids and calcium particles covering lipid pool (LP). M: media. The lipid pool is surrounded by a calcium armor (c). ×100. **D:** fibrous cap. ×400. **E:** Ag stain. Degenerated or disrupted collagen fibers in the superficial layer of extremely thin fibrous cap (arrows). **E:** EVG stain. No elastic fibers in the cap. **F:** Tiel-Nielzen stain. Ceroids (purple) in the cap (arrows). ×400.

Fig. 7. A: angioscopy. Glistening yellow plaque (arrows) with a delle (arrowhead). **B:** IVUS. Low echoic plaque (arrowhead) corresponding to the plaque in A accompanied by calcification arrowhead-like in configuration (arrow). **C:** oil red O and hematoxylin stain. Lipid-rich and loose fibrous cap. x100. LP: lipid pool. C: calcium. M: media. **D:** same fibrous cap. ×400. **E:** Azan stain. Arrowhead: a small perforation in the extremely thin fibrous cap, which corresponds to the delle in panel A. Arrow: bleeding within the plaque. **F:** Ag stain. Arrowhead: a small disruption in fibrous cap composed of residues of atrophied collagen fibers. **G:** fluorescence (yellow) of ceroids in the plaque. ×100.

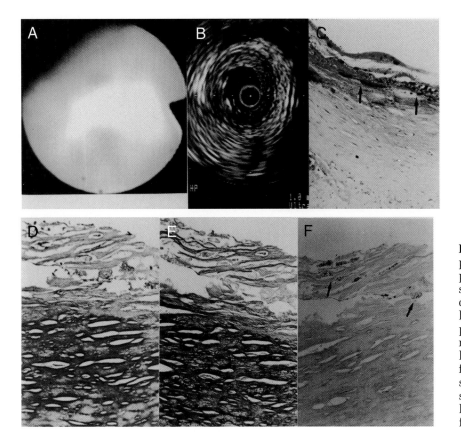

Fig. 8. A: angioscopy. Glistening yellow plaque. **B:** IVUS. Iso- to low echoic plaque. **C:** oil red O and hematoxylin stain. Deposition of lipids and small calcium particles (arrows) in superficial layers of a fibrous plaque without lipid pool inside. ×100. **D:** Ag stain. Atrophic collagen fibers in the superficial layer and tight and dense collagen fibers in deeper layers. **E:** EVG stain absent in elastic fibers. **F:** Tiel-Nielzen stain. Ceroid deposition in superficial layer (arrows). Superficial layer was deformed during slicing. ×400.

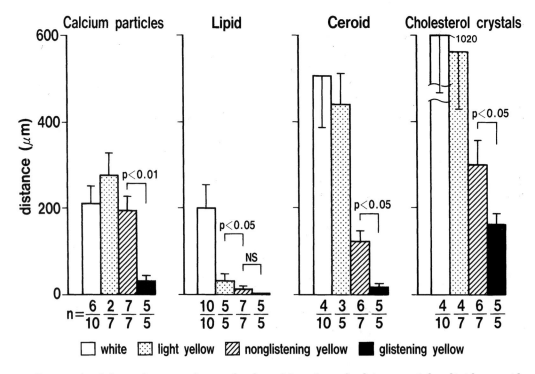

Fig. 9. Shortest distance (μm) from plaque surface to the deposition sites of calcium particles, lipids, ceroids, and cholesterol crystals in lipid pool plaques.

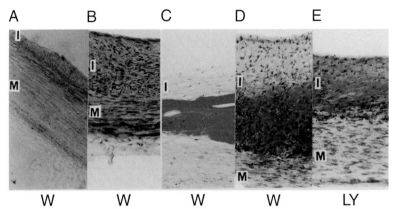

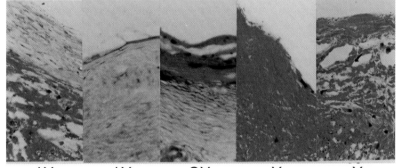

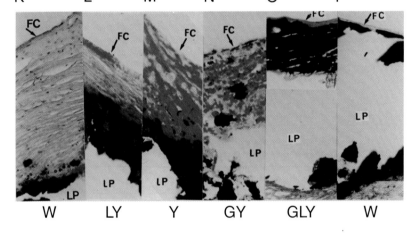

Fig. 10. Various deposition patterns of lipids in the coronary plaques and their relation to surface color by angioscopy. **A:** almost normal coronary segment. I: intima; M: media. **B:** intimal thickening with collagen fiber increase. **C–P:** various deposition patterns of lipids in the plaques. W: white. LY: light yellow. Y: yellow. GY: glistening yellow. GLY: glistening light yellow. FC: fibrous cap. LP: lipid pool.

layer. Collagen fibers in this superficial layer are loose, but they are tight in the deeper layers, and depositions of fine calcium particles and ceroids are also restricted to the superficial layer, indicating that the superficial layer is vulnerable. In in-vitro studies of human coronary arteries removed from sudden coronary death patients, Farb observed plaque erosion without rupture.[5] Whether the superficial type in our study corresponds to that observed by Farb remains to be clarified. It became evident that elastic fibers are deficient and collagen fibers are scarce and degenerated, fragmented, or atrophied in glistening

yellow plaques of the lipid pool type and that similar changes are observed in the superficial layers in nonlipid pool plaque.

The radial distance from the plaque surface to the deposited portions of various substances were examined. It was revealed that in glistening yellow plaques, fine calcium crystals, lipids, and ceroids were deposited close to the surface (Figs. 9), suggesting that these substances reflected illumination showing glistening yellow surfaces.

Fig. 10 shows various histological changes in the plaques and their relation to angioscopic surface color. Thus, it is concluded that glistening yellow plaque is vulnerable (fragile or unstable) and it is composed of 2 subtypes: namely, lipid pool and superficial types. Theoretically, a large disruption extending into the lipid pool can be induced in the former, and superficial disruption, namely erosion, can be induced in the latter. Although definite evidence is lacking, there is a possibility that occlusive thrombus is more easily formed on the former type of plaque. It is necessary to clarify whether acute myocardial infarction develops more often in the former and unstable angina in the latter.

In-Vitro Angioscopic Characterization of Glistening Yellow Plaques

Irrespective of surface color, any intact plaques reflect illumination when output of the light guide of the angioscope is excessively large. Yellow plaques are classified by shape into protruding and nonprotruding (concave or lined). Both categories of plaques reflect illumination when the light guide is close to the plaque or output is too large. When output is decreased or the light guide becomes distant, the majority of plaques cease to glisten. However, there is a specific plaque that continues to glisten like a firefly or a yellow fluorescent substance. The plaques are usually protruded (convex) into the lumen and glisten entirely, or partially at the rim (yellow). These plaques are called "glistening yellow plaques" in our laboratories.

The Nature of Glistening

The atheromatous masses exposed by peeling off the superficial layer still glisten. Histologically, small calcium crystals are disseminated in the lipid-rich masses. On the other hand, in nonglistening and protruding yellow plaque the exposed atheromatous masses do not glisten. Histologically, calcium crystals are not observed in the exposed lipid layers.

It is well known that calcium crystals and cholesterol crystals (both solid and liquid) usually exist in atheromatous plaques.[6] Therefore, in order to confirm whether calcium and cholesterol crystals reflect illumination, microcrystals of $CaHCO_3$ and cholesterol were included in a liquid cholesterol pool previously stained in yellow with beta-carotene. Both crystals glistened in yellow, reflecting illumination.

These findings strongly suggest that small calcium and cholesterol crystals in the superficial layers play a major role in glistening by reflecting illumination through a thin endothelial layer. However, since solid cholesterol crystals are deposited in deeper layers than calcium crystals, it is more likely that calcium crystals play the major role in glistening. Whether other substances including ceroids and liquid calcium crystals[6] glisten remains to be elucidated (Table 1).

Table 1
Coronary Plaque Color and Its Histological Correlations

Angioscopy	Histology							
	Superficial layers (100 μm>)				Mid to deep layers (100 μm<)			
	CF	LIP	CaP	CE	CF	LIP	CaA	CE
1. Nonlipid pool plaques								
White	3+	—	—	—	3+	~1+	—	~1+
Light yellow	3+	1+	—	—	3+	1~2+	—	~1+
Nonglistening yellow	1~2+	3+	—	~1+	1~2+	~3+	—	~1+
Glistening yellow	~1+	3+	+	+	3+	~3+	—	~1+
2. Lipid pool plaques								
White	3+	—	—	—	~1+	1+	~1+	1+
Light yellow	2+	1+	—	—	~1+	1+	~1+	1+
Nonglistening yellow	1~2+	3+	—	~1+	~1+	1+	~1+	1+
Glistening yellow	~1+	3+	1+	1+	—	1+	~1+	1+

CF: collagen fibers; LIP: lipids; CaP: calcium particles; CE: ceroids; CaA: calcium armor around the lipid pool.

—: absent. 1+: slight, or a few. 2+: intermediate. 3+: rich.

Histological Basis for Identification of Calcium Deposition by Angioscopy and IVUS

Limitations of Angioscopy for Detection of Calcium

Calcium crystals can be identified by angioscopy only when they are exposed in the lumen, while IVUS can detect even those in deeper layers, and therefore the latter is superior to the former in detecting calcium deposition.[7-9]

Fig. 11A-C shows a light yellow plaque and small-edged protrusions into the lumen. They reflect illumination in light yellow to grayish in color. IVUS of the same plaque revealed small high echoic spots without shadow in the superficial layer. Histological examination revealed small calcium particles exposed in the lumen.

Fig. 11D-F shows a glistening white mass at the top of a yellow plaque. By IVUS, a thick and high echoic plate with shadowing behind was observed in the superficial layer. This plate is interpreted as calcium. However, due to shadowing, no information on the structure behind was obtainable. Histological examination revealed a large lipid pool surrounded by a calcium armor and it was partially exposed in the lumen through a thin lipid-rich superficial layer. Thus, unless exposed into the lumen, calcium cannot be identified by angioscopy.

Limitations of IVUS for Detection of Calcium

Histologically, calcium is classified into solid and amorphous types, by its shape into small particles, plate-like, nodular, needle-like, and cloud-like, and by its deposition sites into superficial, middle, deep, and disseminated. It is generally believed that calcium is accompanied by echo shadowing. However, there is a limitation to IVUS in identifying calcium.

Using a 30-MHz IVUS probe, Peters concluded that sensitivity and specificity for calcium are 77% and 100%, respectively, and calcium less than 250 μm in diameter cannot be discriminated.[9]

In addition, amorphous (noncrystalized) calcium deposition leads to misinterpretation. When deposited in lipid-rich plaque, it exhibits a high echoic plaque by IVUS (Fig. 12).

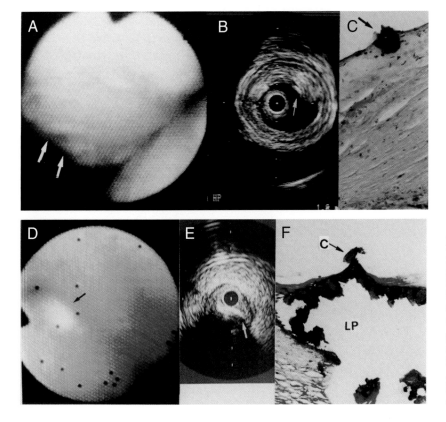

Fig. 11. Exposed calcium particles into the lumen. **A:** angioscopy. Glistening light yellow small protrusions (arrows). **B:** IVUS. A high echoic mass without shadowing in the superficial layer (arrow). **C:** oil red O and hematoxylin stain. A calcium particle exposed in the lumen (arrow). ×400. **D:** angioscopy. A glistening grayish white mass exposed into the lumen (arrow). **E:** IVUS image. **F:** oil red O and hematoxylin stain. A part of calcium armor exposed into the lumen (arrow C). ×100. LP: lipid pool. C: calcium.

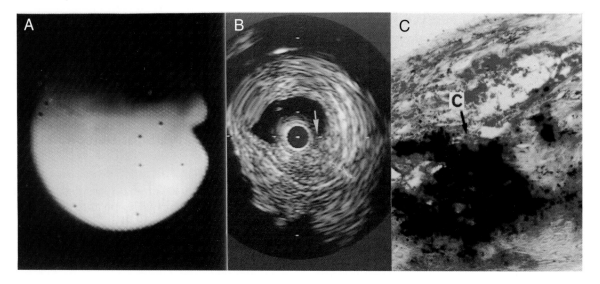

Fig. 12. A: angioscopy. A nonglistening yellow plaque (arrow). **B:** IVUS. A high echoic eccentric plaque without shadowing, which corresponds to that in A. **C:** oil red O and hematoxylin stain. Cloud-like deposition of calcium (probably noncrystallized; arrow c). ×100.

Calcium in the coronary plaques is not necessarily accompanied by echo shadowing behind it. Also, identification of solid calcium is dependent on size and coaxial distance (depth) from the plaque surface. When a 30-MHz conventional IVUS probe was used, calcium particles within 50 μm, within 100 μm, and within 500 μm in maximum diameter, respectively, located within 100 μm, 100 to 500 μm, and over 500 μm in depth were not identified. Furthermore, amor-

phous calcium deposition up to 250 μm in diameter was rarely detectable by conventional IVUS (Fig. 13). Therefore, a lipid-rich and collagen fiber-deficient, namely vulnerable, plaque with deposition of amorphous calcium or disseminated small calcium crystals may be misinterpreted as a fibrotic plaque, since it may apparently exhibit a high echoic plaque without shadowing. Thus, it should be noted that a high echoic plaque does not necessarily mean a stable

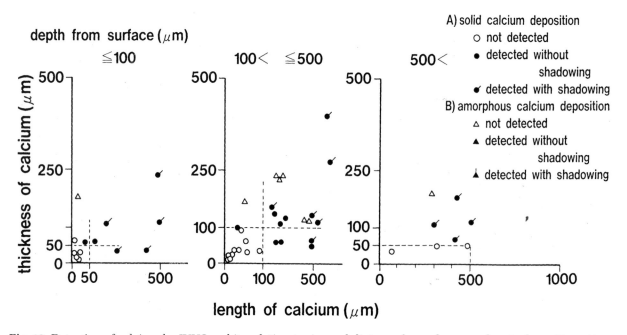

Fig. 13. Detection of calcium by IVUS and its relation to size and distance from plaque surface to deposition sites.

plaque. Also, it has been pointed out that fibrotic plaques may exhibit high echoic plaques with shadowing.[8,9]

Histological Basis for Detection of a Lipid Pool by IVUS

Angioscopy and angiography are not suited for observation of a lipid pool within the coronary plaques. The sole clinically applicable method for detection of a lipid pool is IVUS.

It is generally believed that regions of a lipid pool (core) are identified as large echolucent areas within the plaque and are distinguished from calcium-induced echo dropout because the echolucent lipid pool is surrounded centrally and peripherally by tissue reflections. However, a lipid pool does not necessarily exhibit a uniform low echoic area due to calcium deposition. Because it is frequently wrapped with a thick calcium armor and hidden by echo shadowing, it is frequently difficult to distinguish the lipid pool from echo dropout. Therefore, identifica-

tion of its existence by calcium deposition patterns should be established.

The ultrasonographic images related to the lipid pool shown in Fig. 14 correspond to histological changes shown in Fig. 15, and they are schematically shown in Fig. 16. A high echoic smooth line up to 0.3 mm in width in superficial and one up to 0.2 mm in a deep layer in known to reflect internal and external elastic lamina, respectively (panel A in Figs. 14, 15, and 16). High echoic spots in the low echoic middle layer may indicate a lipid pool (Figs. 14B, 15A,B, and 16B). A high echoic plate over 0.3 mm in thickness in a superficial layer, irrespective of the presence or absence of shadowing behind, strongly suggests a lipid pool beneath (Figs. 14C,D, 15D, 16C,D). A uniform low echoic area with or without a high echoic plate behind it indicates that it is a lipid pool (Figs. 14E,J, 15E1,I,J, 16E,J). High echoic thick plates in both superficial and deep layers indicate a lipid pool between them (Figs. 14F,H, 15E2,H, 16F,H). Also, thick and irregular high echoic plates, sometimes arrowhead-like, in the middle layer indicate a lipid pool in the adjacent areas (Figs. 14G,I, 15F,G, 16G,I).

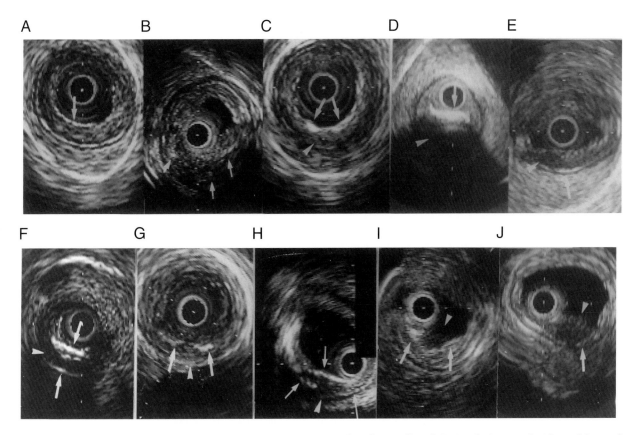

Fig. 14. Various deposition patterns of calcium by IVUS (arrows of each panel) and their relations to lipid pool (arrowhead of each panel). Alphabet letters correspond respectively to those in Figs. 15 and 16.

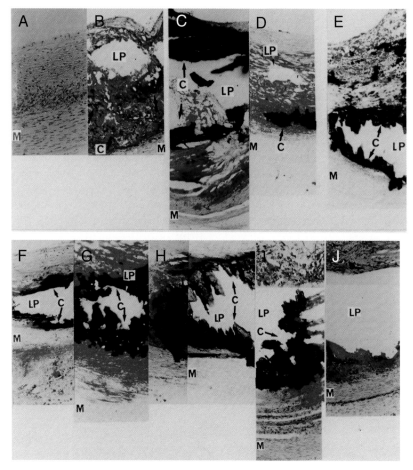

Fig. 15. Various localizations of lipid pool (LP) and their relation to calcium (C) deposition.

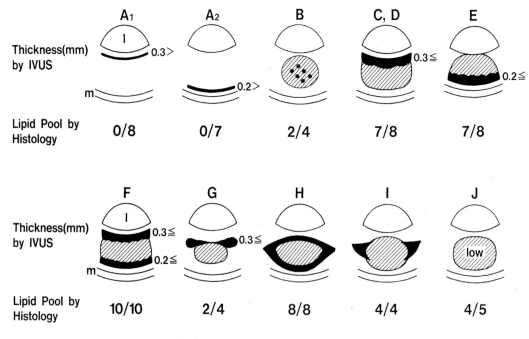

m:media, l:lumen, shaded area : lipid pool by histology

Fig. 16. Schematic representation of a lipid pool and its relation to calcium deposition patterns reconstructed based on Figs. 14 and 15. Incidence of lipid pool identified histologically in each calcium distribution patterns.

References

1. Sherman CT, Litvack F, Grundfest W, et al: Coronary angioscopy in patients with unstable angina pectoris. N Engl J Med 315:913–919, 1986.
2. Uchida Y, Tomaru T, Nakamura F, et al: Percutaneous coronary angioscopy in patients with ischemic heart disease. Am Heart J 114:1069–1075, 1989.
3. Lillie RD: Histopathologic Technique and Practical Histochemistry. 4th ed. McGraw Hill, NY, 1976, pp 533–543.
4. Maeda T: Ceroid staining. In: New Histochemistry. 3rd ed. Asakura Publishing Co., Tokyo, 1980, pp 630–653.
5. Farb A, Burke AP, Tang AL, et al: Coronary plaque erosion without rupture into a lipid core. Circulation 93:1354–1363, 1996.
6. Amanuma K: Studies on fine structure and location of lipids in quick-freeze replicas of atherosclerotic aorta of WHHL rabbits. Virchows Arch A410:231–238, 1986.
7. Gussenhoven EJ, Essed CE, Lancee CT, et al: Arterial wall characteristics determined by intravascular ultrasound imaging: An in vitro study. J Am Coll Cardiol 14:947–952, 1989.
8. Tobis JM, Mallery JA, Mahon D, et al: Intravascular ultrasound imaging of human coronary arteries in vivo: Analysis of tissue characterizations with comparison to histological specimens. Circulation 83:913–926, 1991.
9. Peters RJG, Kok WEM, Havenith MG, et al: Histopathologic validation of intracoronary ultrasound imaging. J Am Soc Echocardiogr 7:230–241, 1994.

Chapter 6

Relationships Between Angioscopic Images and Histological Changes of Complex Plaques

"Complex" means "disruption of any forms and degrees." Endothelial damage is microscopically "complex." However, unless significantly extensive, its identification is beyond conventional angioscopy and IVUS. In addition, it may be induced simply by insertion of angioscopes and IVUS probes themselves and even by floppy guidewires. Therefore, the plaques with minimal endothelial damage are not included in "complex plaques" in the present classification. Fig. 1 shows a representative example of a disrupted plaque that was found in the anterior descending coronary artery (LAD) in a patient who died in an ambulance 2 hours after the onset of chest pain. Angioscopically, the plaque was a fractured yellow plaque with a red thrombus on it. Histologically, the plaque had a large lipid pool inside; a thin fibrous cap was ruptured at a rim, and an occlusive thrombus mixed with atheromatous debris was formed on it.

Clinically, it is generally believed that the angiographically most stenotic segment is the culprit for acute coronary syndromes. However, this is not always the case. Figs.2A and 2B show a removed coronary segment in which the plaque at the most stenotic portion was intact and a plaque located in a portion proximal to the most stenotic segment was disrupted. This indicates the importance of a survey of the proximal less stenotic segments.

Fig. 3 shows bleeding in a white plaque of a coronary segment that was removed from a patient who died of acute myocardial infarction. By IVUS, a uniformly high echoic area was observed in the superficial to middle layers of a concentric plaque. Histologically, a hematoma was found in a collagen fiber-rich layer without lipid deposition.

Fig. 4 shows a localized defect (ulcer) of yellow plaque with exposed yellow matter. By IVUS, a defect in a concentric plaque was found close to a superficial calcification. Histologically, the bottom of the defect was composed of exposed lipids and calcium particles. Whether such a histological change is common to the ulcers clinically observed is unclear.

Fig. 5 shows a membranous, yellow, transparent mass observed in a patient who died of acute myocardial infarction. Histologically, the mass was not a part of atherosclerotic plaque but a fibrin-rich mass. It was likely a remnant of an autolysed thrombus.

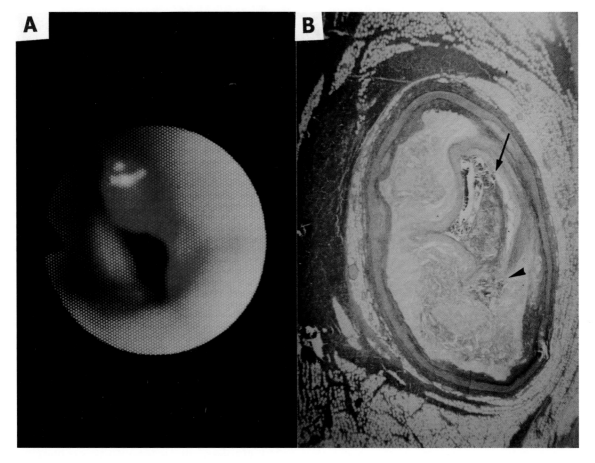

Fig. 1. A disrupted yellow plaque observed in a patient who died 2 hours after the onset of chest pain. **A:** a disrupted plaque with red thrombus. **B:** coaxial section of the same plaque. A large lipid pool, rupture at a rim where the fibrous cap was very thin, and a thrombus mixed with atheromatous tissue on it.

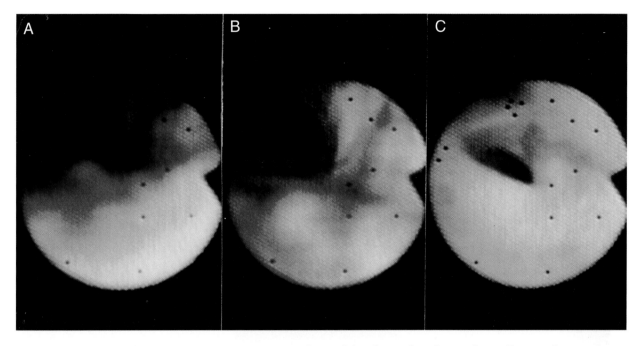

Fig. 2A. A disruption in a less stenotic portion. **A:** proximal rim of the plaque that glistened in yellow. **B:** disrupted portion covered with a red thrombus. **C:** the most stenotic portion just distal to the disrupted portion.

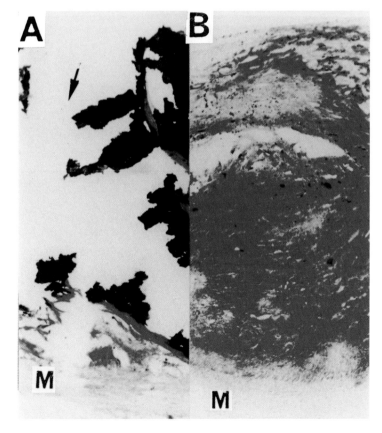

Fig. 2B. Histological changes of the plaques, same as those in Fig. 2A. **A:** the disrupted portion. A vacant lipid pool and destructed surrounding calcium armor. **B:** the most stenotic portion. M: media.

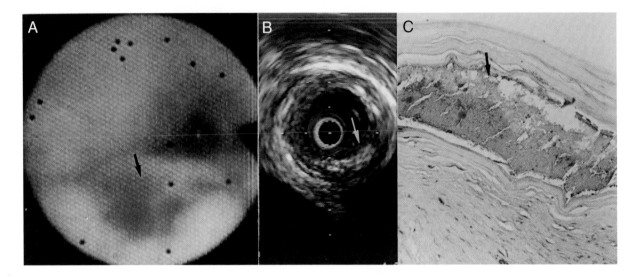

Fig. 3. A: Angioscopy. Bleeding in a yellow plaque. **B:** IVUS. A homogenous high echoic area. **C:** a hematoma that may correspond to the high echoic area in B.

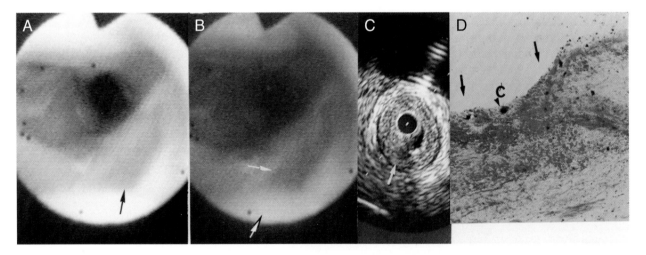

Fig. 4. A: angioscopy. A localized but relatively deep defect (arrow). **B:** dye staining with Evans blue. Portions in blue indicate damaged endothelium. **C:** IVUS. A defect that corresponds to that in A. **D:** oil red O and hematoxylin stain. Arrows: defect. c: calcium particle.

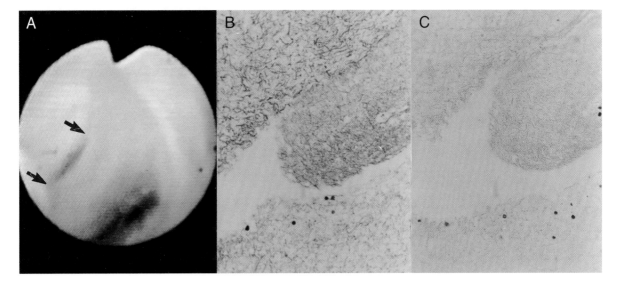

Fig. 5. A: a yellow and transparent membranous mass in a coronary segment. **B:** PTAH stain for fibrin. Blue threads are fibrin. **C:** Giemsa stain for platelets. No platelets.

Chapter 7

Relationships Between Our Angioscopic Classification and Histological Classification Recommended by the AHA Council

White plaque in our study was histologically composed of type III, type Vb, and type Vc. Nonglistening yellow plaque was composed of types IV and Va. Glistening yellow plaque was composed of types IV and Va or Vc with superficial fragility. Thus, angioscopic classification does not completely correspond to that recommended by the AHA Council.[1] Histological study showed that plaque progression is not uniform and seems not to occur as described.

For example, we observed at least 5 types of lipid pools when the character of the fibrous cap and calcium deposition were taken into consideration. The most frequently observed type was a lipid pool with tight calcium armor and a tight, thick fibrous cap. Less frequently observed types were lipid pools with thick fibrous caps, those with lipid with or without calcium armor, and with lipid-deposited collagen-deficient thin fibrous caps. Lipid pools without calcium armor and with lipid-rich and collagen fiber-deficient plaque may correspond to type IV of the AHA classification. However, this type was rare.

Reference

1. Stary HC, Chandler AB, Dinsmore RE, et al: A definition of advanced types of atherosclerotic lesions and a histological classification of atherosclerosis: A report from the Committee on Vascular Lesions of the Council on Arteriosclerosis. American Heart Association. Circulation 92:1355–1374, 1995.

Chapter 8

Histological Basis for Natural Courses Toward Vulnerable Plaques and Disruption:

With Special Reference to Acute Coronary Syndromes

Possible Courses of Plaque Progression

Type IV of the AHA classification is vulnerable, and this type of plaque is covered with collagen and then stabilized, and when it does not occur, it remains vulnerable.[1] However, the time course changes in the identical plaque have never been examined clinically; whether the reverse process occurs remains to be seen.

There are at least 7 possible courses of plaque progression (Fig. 1). In course A, collagen fibers increase in number and remain undamaged and not deposited with lipids, resulting in a large fibrous plaque (Fig. 2).

In course B, lipid deposition occurs at the middle to deep layers of a fibrous plaque preceded or followed by destruction of collagen fibers, and a large lipid pool is formed. However, a thick fibrous cap remains intact and the lipid pool is encapsulated with calcium armor, resulting in a progressed but stable plaque (Fig. $3C_1$), or the collagen fibers are replaced with lipids and calcium particles due to inflammatory, metabolic, and/or mechanical processes, resulting in a vulnerable plaque (Fig. $3C_2$), or a tight calcium armor surrounding the lipid pool is formed just beneath the very thin and fragile cap and acts against large and deep disruption, resulting in a less vulnerable plaque, even though a very thin fibrous cap remains vulnerable and erosion may occur in it (Fig. $3C_3$).

In course C, collagen fibers in all layers are replaced by lipids. Then, lipid pool formation and a collagen fiber-deficient, lipid-rich, and calcium-deposited fragile fibrous cap is formed, resulting in a vulnerable plaque (Fig. 4). Superficial deposition of crystals such as calcium and cholesterol may enhance further destruction by friction with surrounding fragile tissues and also with endothelium, resulting in disruption and occlusive thrombus formation. Deposition of calcium particles may require a considerably long time. Existence of atrophic or fragmented collagen fibers and their remnants in a very thin fibrous cap may support the existence of this process (see Chapter 5).

In course D, a plaque with fragile and loose collagen layers develops at first, followed by lipid deposition and lipid pool formation. Then, a collagen fiber-rich tight fibrous cap is formed, resulting in a stable plaque as described by the AHA Council (Fig. $5D_1$), or it remains as a vulnerable plaque because collagen fiber increase does not occur (Fig. $5D_2$).

In course E, endothelial cells alone or collagen fibers in the superficial layers of the collagen fiber-rich fibrous plaque are damaged by inflammatory, metabolic, and/or mechanical processes, resulting in a vulnerable plaque of a superficial type (Fig. 6).

Whether all of these courses actually occur in a clinical situation is not known. Also, which category of these courses a given plaque chooses is not known.

51

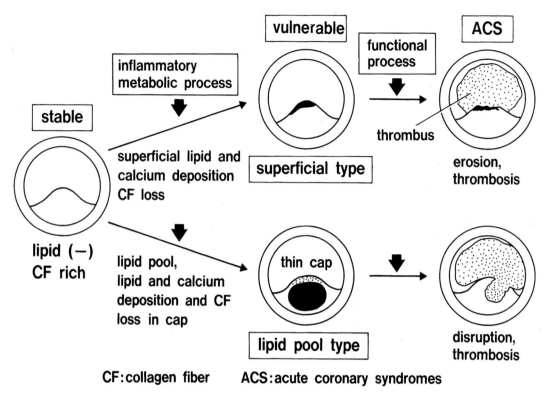

Fig. 1. Possible processes toward birth of vulnerable plaque.

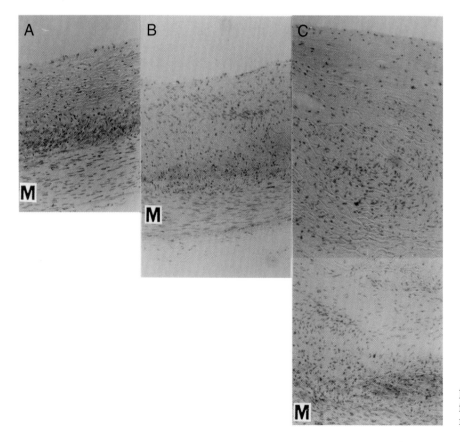

Fig. 2. Growth of a fibrous (collagen fiber-rich) plaque from A toward C. Almost no deposition of lipids.

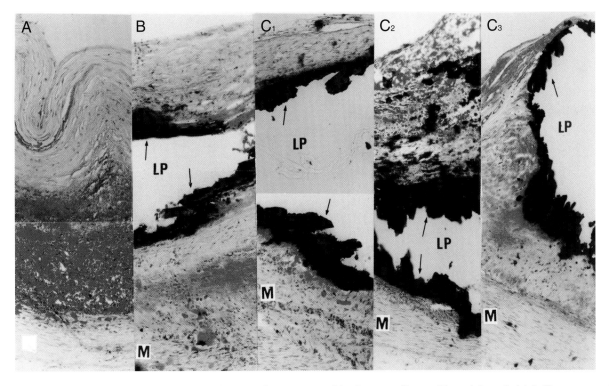

Fig. 3. Progression of a fibrous plaque to 3 different plaques. **B:** stable due to collagen fiber-rich and thick fibrous cap. **C₁:** increase in size of lipid pool (LP) and thinning of fibrous cap but still stable. **C₂:** vulnerable due to collagen fiber loss and deposition of lipids and calcium particles. **C₃:** a tight calcium armor located just beneath a thin fibrous cap. The superficial layer may be vulnerable but the armor may act against large disruption. M: media.

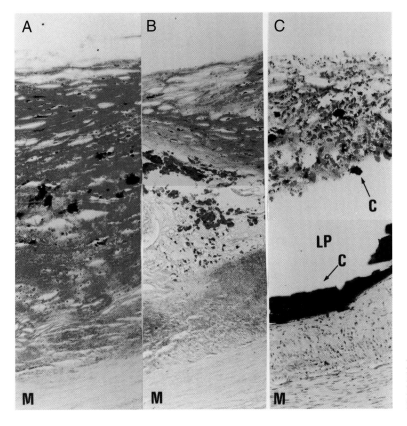

Fig. 4. Diffuse deposition of lipids followed by lipid pool C: calcium. M: media. formation and loss of collagen fibers in the fibrous cap, resulting in a vulnerable plaque.

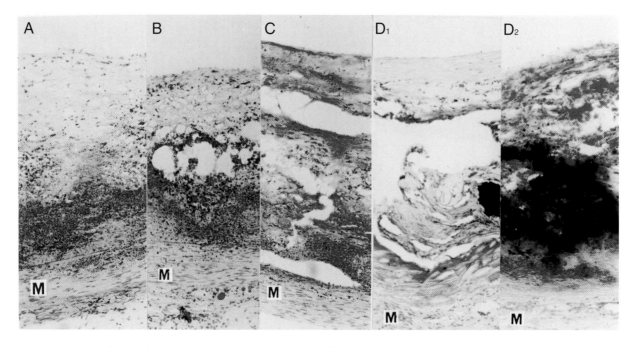

Fig. 5. Formation of a loose plaque composed of fragile collagen fibers at first (**A**), followed by lipid deposition and cavity formation due to deposition of liquid lipid (**B, C**). **D₁**: new formation of collagen fiber-rich fibrous cap and the plaque becomes stable. **D₂**: further deposition of lipids and calcium, and loss of collagen fibers, resulting in a vulnerable plaque. M: media.

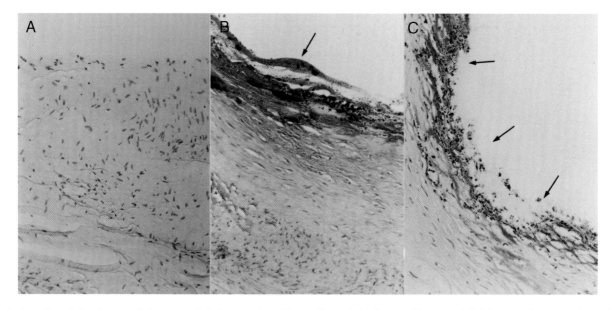

Fig. 6. A vulnerable plaque of the superficial type. **A:** collagen fiber-rich plaque. **B:** superficial layers alone are deposited with lipids and calcium particles, and collagen fibers are lost. **C:** formation of an erosion in the superficial layer (arrows).

Plaque Disruption and Its Relation to Acute Coronary Syndromes

Fig. 7 shows possible processes toward acute coronary syndromes proposed by Fuster[2] and mod-

ified by us. Disruption of a vulnerable plaque with a lipid pool inside results in immediate thrombus formation on it. The atheromatous debris in the pool may be ejected into the lumen and form a mixture with thrombus, or flow downstream, or remain inside. When the thrombus occludes the lumen com-

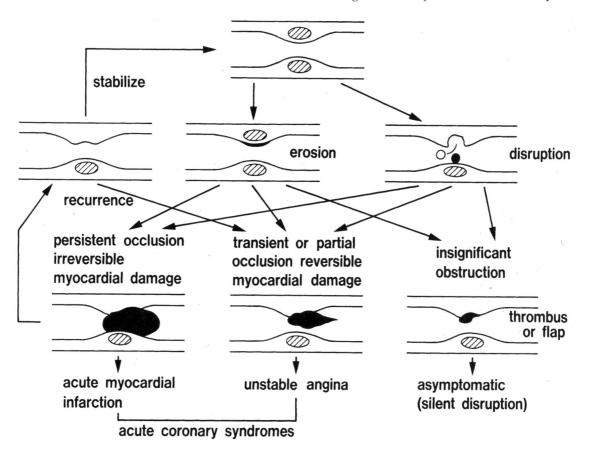

Fig. 7. Schematic representation of plaque disruption and thrombosis, and their relation to different coronary syndromes. Used with permission from ref. 2 and partially modified.

pletely for a long time, irreversible myocardial damage, namely acute myocardial infarction, develops. When, the thrombus occludes the lumen completely but transiently, severe myocardial ischemia but with reversible myocardial damage occurs, resulting in unstable angina pectoris. The same processes may occur in vulnerable plaques of the superficial type in which only superficial disruption likely occurs. Whether this type is more related to unstable angina is not known. When a significant reduction in coronary blood flow does not occur, the patient is asymptomatic, and therefore this situation is called "silent disruption." Sudden cardiac

death due to ischemia-related ventricular arrhythmias may develop following disruption in a certain group of patients. Therefore, it is also included in acute coronary syndromes.

Rheologically, reducing fibrous cap thickness increases peak circumferential wall stress in the plaque whereas increasing severity of stenosis decreases peak stress in the plaque.[3] Therefore, a thin and fragile fibrous cap and increased intraluminal pressure in combination further accelerate plaque disruption. This rheological mechanism may be another reason for disruption of the plaques in coronary segments with insignificant stenosis.

References

1. Stary HC, Chandler AB, Dinsmore RE, et al: A definition of advanced types of atherosclerotic lesions and a histological classification of atherosclerosis: A report from the Committee on Vascular Lesions of the Council on Arteriosclerosis. American Heart Association Circulation 92:1355–1374, 1995.

2. Fuster V, Badimon L: The pathogenesis of coronary artery disease and the acute coronary syndromes. N Engl J Med 326:242–250, 1992.

3. Loree HM, Kamm RD, Stringfellow RG, Lee RT: Effects of fibrous cap thickness on circumferential stress in model atherosclerotic vessels. Circ Res 71:850–858, 1992.

Chapter 9

Physiological and Histological Basis for Understanding Bloodstream, Vascular Endothelial Cell Damage, Thrombosis, and Thrombolysis

Angioscopic and Angiomicroscopic Basis for Understanding Bloodstream in the Coronary Artery

Bloodstream in the Stenotic Native Artery

Rheologically, it is well known that the modality of blood flow has a keen relation to thrombus formation. Therefore, it is important to have enough knowledge of blood flow in the nonstenotic and stenotic coronary arteries for understanding the underlying mechanisms for thrombosis and thrombolysis. Clinically, we can observe it from upstream by angioscopy. However, insertion of an angioscope itself may greatly modify the bloodstream. Therefore, observation from downstream is necessary to understand the natural bloodstream. Clinically, however, it is difficult for conventional angioscopy to observe the bloodstream from downstream.

To get insight into the bloodstream in nonstenotic as well as in stenotic coronary arteries, the canine iliac artery perfused with Krebs-Henseleit solution and pulsatile backflow from a renal artery was drained into the perfusion circuit to produce a laminal bloodstream, and it was observed from downstream by either a conventional angioscope or an angiomicroscope.[1] Also, isolated human coronary artery was perfused for observation of the bloodstream from downstream.[2]

In nonstenotic arteries, the bloodstream was usually composed of a central main stream (coaxial stream) that ran along the central longitudinal axis, and peripheral streams that ran beside the longitudi-

nal axis. Both types of streams rotated along the longitudinal axis clockwise or counterclockwise during systole. When the constriction exceeded 50%, the peripheral streams rotated along the outlet of the stenotic segment, causing curls toward the minor axis (Fig. 1A–C). In addition, the outer layers of the coaxial stream were separated and turned upstream, causing longitudinal curls. When the constriction exceeded 75%, the coaxial stream splayed at the outlet of the stenotic segment and thereafter became obscure, while the peripheral streams rotated around the outlet, causing one or more curls to develop.

In the segments just beneath the bifurcation, the peripheral bloodstream turned upstream. In the coronary artery of the beating heart, the modality of the bloodstream may be far more complex due to systolic and diastolic pulsatile flows that are modified by curves and stenoses.[3,4]

Fig. 2 shows the bloodstream in stents implanted in the canine iliac artery. Irrespective of the types of stents used clinically for dilatation of the coronary artery, blood turbulence occurred. Blood flow turbulence became more marked when stent dilatation was insufficient.

Relationships Between the Bloodstream and Thrombosis

Without stenosis in the human coronary perfusion model, thin thrombi scattered on the luminal surface; however, they did not grow into large thrombi. With stenosis, a thin thrombus appeared along the minor axis curls of the bloodstream at the outlet of stenosis. The thrombus grew gradually to a globular shape, or into doughnut-like shape (Fig. 1D–F).

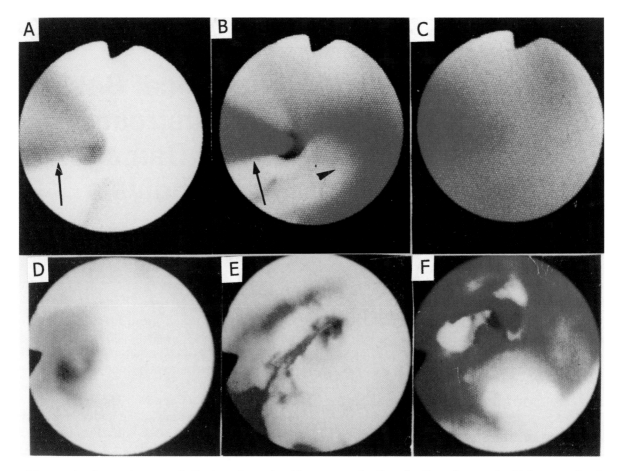

Fig. 1. Observation by angioscopy. **A–C:** stenotic canine iliac artery. **A:** diastole. **B:** early systole. **C:** late systole. Arrows in A and B: coaxial stream. Arrowheads in B: curling peripheral stream. **D–F:** isolated stenotic human coronary artery. **A:** before blood perfusion. **E:** 5 min after blood perfusion. **F:** 10 min after blood perfusion. Used with permission from refs. 1 and 2.

Also, thrombi appeared at the center of longitudinal curls and grew into globular shapes.[1] Just beneath the bifurcation, a thrombus was frequently formed at the center of the backward curls (Fig. 3). These bloodstream-related thrombus formations may also occur clinically in the stenotic coronary artery. The thrombus thus formed remains not innocent. It acts to disperse the bloodstream further to accelerate thrombus formation.

Angiomicroscopic and Histological Basis for Discrimination of Damaged Endothelial Cells

Identification of vascular endothelial cell damage is extremely important since these cells protect the vessel wall against thrombosis and invasion of various substances and cells. However, conventional angioscopy cannot discriminate between intact and damaged (dead) endothelial cells. To discriminate damaged endothelial cells, we used Evans blue dye, which is generally used for identification of dead culture cells in vitro[5,6] and confirmed its applicability in vivo.[7]

We call this new diagnostic method "dye image angioscopy" or "dye image angiomicroscopy." Various dyes that can stain the human coronary artery are listed in Table 1. Except for Evans blue, safety has not been confirmed for the other dyes.

Animal Experiments

Fig. 4A shows apparently intact canine common iliac artery perfused with Krebs-Henseleit solution. Immediately after bolus injection of 0.2 mL of 5% Evans blue solution into the perfusion circuit, multiple longitudinal strips blue in color were brought about (Fig. 4B). Light microscopic examination re-

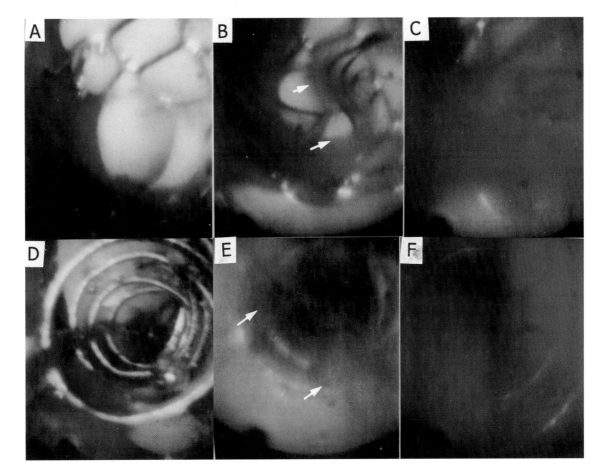

Fig. 2. Angiomicroscopic study. Bloodstream in the stented artery. **A–C:** MultiLink stent. **B:** blood turbulence (arrows). **C:** complete dispersion of blood stream by increasing flow velocity. **D–G:** Giantigo-Roubin II stent. **E:** blood turbulence (arrows). **F:** bloodstream dispersion.

vealed exfoliated endothelial cells and internal elastic lamina (Fig. 4C). Transmission electron microscopy revealed vacuolization in and/or exfoliation of the endothelial cells (Fig. 4E).

Removed Human Coronary Artery

Removed atherosclerotic human coronary segment was also stained with this dye. Fig. 5A shows a yellow plaque with apparently smooth surface even by angiomicroscopy. After Evans blue, however, multiple blue portions were brought about (Fig. 5B). These portions fluttered or vibrated during perfusion. Light microscopy revealed that these stained portions were exfoliated endothelial cells (Fig. 5C).

Also, it was revealed that yellow layers beneath the endothelial cells were collagen fibers with lipid deposition and they were not stained (Fig. 5D). Furthermore, the exposed atheromatous tissues were not stained with this dye.

Angiomicroscopic and Histological Basis for Thrombosis and Thrombolysis

Discrimination of Thrombus Composition

The effects of thrombolytic therapy are greatly influenced by the composition of the thrombus. Theoretically, a thrombus composed mainly of platelets is resistant to thrombolytic agents. That composed mainly of red blood cells with loose fibrin network is susceptible to thrombolytic agents. Therefore, it is clinically important to discriminate thrombus composition.

An artificial thrombus was made and various dyes were added under light microscopy; it was revealed that fibrin is stained in blue with Evans blue and platelets are stained in dark purple by a combi-

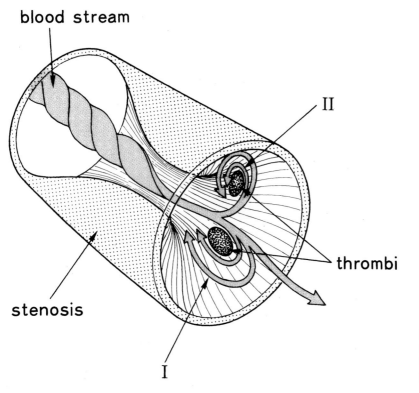

blood stream

II

thrombi

stenosis

I

Fig. 3. Schematic representation of the blood-stream in the stenotic artery and its relation to thrombus formation. I: coaxial curl. II: longitudinal curl.

nation of Evans blue and eosin (Fig. 6). Dyes that can stain thrombus are listed in Table 2. However, except Evans blue, the safety of these stains for clinical use has not been confirmed.

Process of Thrombus Birth and Growth

Animal Experiments

When endothelium is damaged or exfoliated, thrombus formation occurs within several seconds. It is generally believed that platelet adhesion onto the damaged endothelium or tissues beneath occurs first,

and then other blood cells and fibrin are attached, forming a red thrombus.

Fig. 7 shows the processes of growth of a globular thrombus. A thin mural thrombus appeared first, then protruded thrombus developed, and finally a globular thrombus was formed. This process usually occurs within 10 minutes in dogs.

During growth, multiple fibrin threads extended from the thrombus surface, and blood corpuscles were trapped by the threads. This process was repeated and a large globular thrombus was finally formed (Fig. 8). This finding gives us an important insight as to how to prevent thrombus growth (Fig. 9).

Table 1
Staining of Cells and Substances Composing Human Coronary Artery

| Dyes | EC | | VSMC | IEL | CF | EF | FC |
	live	dead					
Evans blue	—	+	—	—	—	—	—
Eosin	—	—	—	+	—	—	—
Fucsin	—	—	—	+	+	+	—
Sudan black	—	—	—	—	—	—	+

EC: endothelial cells. VSMC: vascular smooth muscle cells. IEL: internal elastic lamina. CF: collagen fiber. EF: elastic fiber. FC: foam cells.

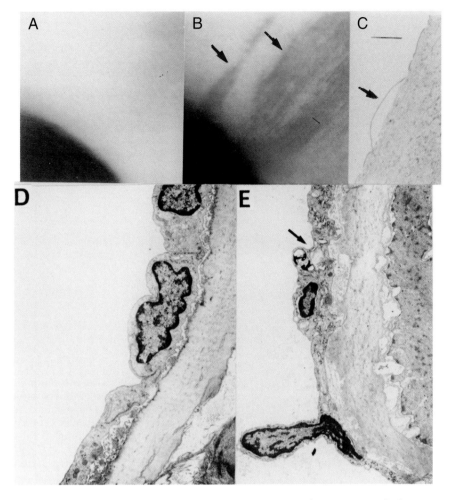

Fig. 4. Angiomicroscopic features of luminal surface of a canine common iliac artery. **A:** before Evans blue dye. **B:** immediately after the dye. Arrows: damaged endothelial cells stained in blue. **C:** light microscopic changes in the same artery. Arrow: exfoliated endothelial cells and internal elastic lamina. Horizontal bar: 100 μm. Transmission electron microscopic features of intact (**D**) and damaged endothelial cells (**E**). Arrow in E: vacuolization of endothelial cell.

Isolated and Perfused Human Coronary Artery

Figs. 10A and B shows thrombus formation in an isolated human coronary artery by perfusing canine arterial blood.[2] The artery had an ulcer on a plaque. After blood perfusion, a thrombus was formed around the ulcer but not in the ulcer. Although the surrounding portions were stained, the ulcer itself was not stained with Evans blue, indicating that at least fibrin has no affinity to ulcer and thrombus is not formed in the ulcer (Fig. 10B). Light microscopy of the same plaque revealed that fibrin threads were formed on the endothelium but not on the tissues (collagen fibers) beneath the endothelium, as in canine experiments (Fig. 10D,E).

Based on this finding, it is considered that clinically observed thrombus formed on the disrupted plaque does not arise from the exposed atheromatous tissues and collagen fibers. It probably arises from the damaged endothelium surrounding the disrupted portion and rides on the plaque after growth.

Effects of Washout on Thrombus Appearance

Clinically, saline and contrast materials are generally injected repeatedly into the coronary artery during angiography or interventions. Since affinity to platelets or fibrin is weak, red blood cells may easily be detached, resulting in a thrombus devoid of red blood cells, namely pink to white thrombus.

To confirm this possibility, we observed the process of the changes in color and shape of a thrombus caused by infusion of saline solution. The red

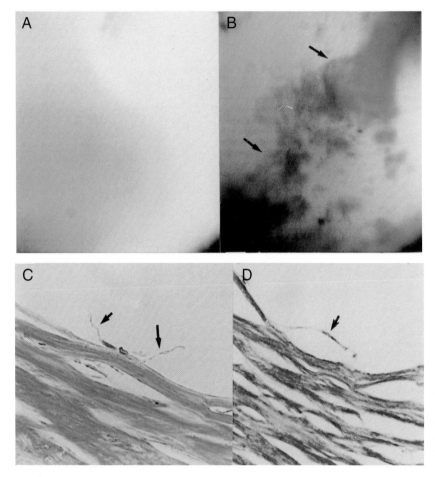

Fig. 5. Isolated human coronary artery. **A:** atherosclerotic segment before Evans blue. **B:** after Evans blue. Arrows: exfoliated endothelial cells. **C:** Azan stain. Arrows: exfoliated endothelial cells. **D:** Ag stain for collagen. Arrow: exfoliated endothelial cells. Purplish brown portion: collagen fibers.

thrombus gradually changed in color into pink within 10 minutes, and then into white within 30 minutes of saline infusion. Thereafter, a bundle-like structure was gradually exposed (Fig. 11). This structure was stained in blue with Evans blue, indicating that it is composed mainly of fibrin. Bridge or web formation clinically observed in the coronary or pulmonary artery may be formed by the same mechanisms.

Frosty Glass-Like Luminal Surface

During blood perfusion, a frosty glass-like surface of the arterial wall is not infrequently observed during blood perfusion in animal artery and in isolated human coronary artery. Also, the same coronary luminal surface is not infrequently observed in patients with acute coronary syndromes (see Chapter 12).

Fig. 12 shows a frosty glass-like surface observed in an isolated human coronary artery induced by saline infusion that was performed following mural thrombus formation. The frosty glass-like surface was stained with Evans blue. Histologically, multiple fibrin threads adhered to blood corpuscles arising from the endothelium were observed. This finding suggests that a frosty glass-like surface in a clinical situation is also caused by the remnant of thrombus after washout and that such a change implies preexisting thrombus.

Process of Thrombolysis

Responses to thrombolytic agents are greatly influenced by the composition and age of the thrombus. In case of globular thrombus, which is usually formed 10 to 30 minutes after blood perfusion in dogs, blood corpuscles are detached from the thrombus surface resembling a sandstorm, and the thrombus surface becomes smooth and its size is gradually reduced (Fig. 13B). Closer observation shows that fibrin threads extending from the thrombus surface are lysed and blood corpuscles attached to them are detached, resulting in a reduction in size. In contrast, in the case of a mural thrombus that was recently formed, small blocks detached from the mother thrombus and

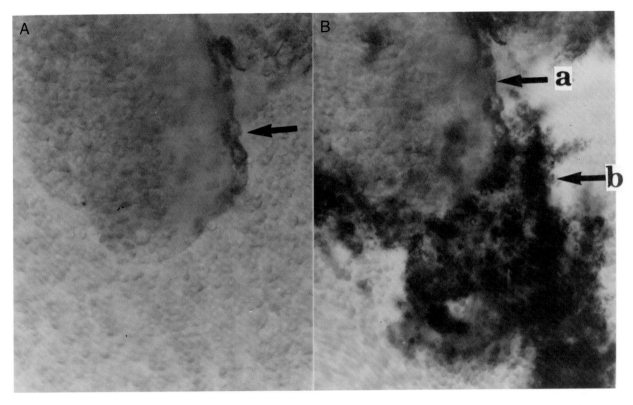

Fig. 6. Dye staining of thrombus. **A:** Evans blue stain. Arrow: fibrin. **B:** Evans blue followed by eosin. Arrow a: fibrin. Arrow b: platelet aggregates.

flowed downstream (Fig. 13C,D). This may be due to regional difference in composition, especially in the fibrin network. Small fibrin or platelet blocks also detached from the globular thrombus when it became very small, or the steal that connected it to the vessel wall was lysed. Thus, we should know that there are 2 modalities of thrombosis: dispersion into blood cells and division into small blocks, and that the latter may again induce distal occlusion, resulting in a no re-flow phenomenon and/or infarction (Fig. 14).

Therefore, the latter phenomenon is not a true lysis. Thrombolytic agents that do not cause such an unwanted phenomenon are required.

Ultrasound Thrombolysis: A Future Technology

Ultrasound irradiation through the chest wall accelerates coronary thrombolysis with tPA. It is con-

Table 2
Dye Staining of Thrombus

Dye	Fibrin	Platelet	White Blood Cell	Red Blood Cell
Evans blue	blue	—	—	—
Eosin	—	red	red	—
Evans blue + Eosin	blue	dark purple	—	—
Fucsin	—	purple	—	—
Fucsin + Evans blue	blue	blue	—	blue
Gentian violet	purple	purple	—	—
Gentian violet + Eosin	dark purple	blue	—	—

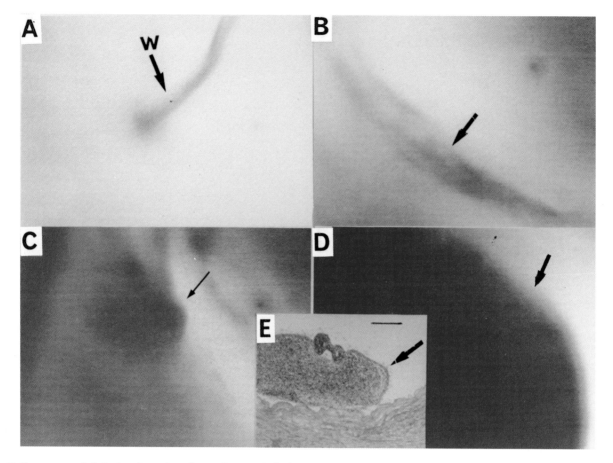

Fig. 7. Processes of globular thrombus formation. **A–C:** before, 5, 10, and 30 minutes after blood perfusion, respectively. **E:** Light microscopic changes of the same thrombus. W in A: a stainless steel wire 70 μm in diameter.

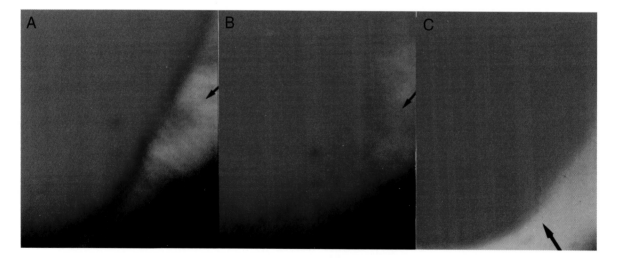

Fig. 8. Fine structure of thrombus growth. **A:** fibrin threads extending outward (arrow). **B:** adhesion of blood corpuscles on the threads (arrow). **C:** increased size of the thrombus.

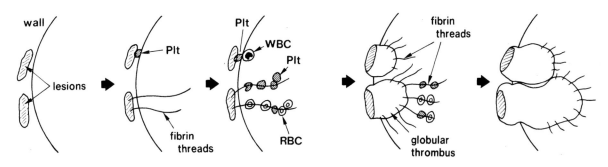

Fig. 9. Schematic representation of the processes of thrombus birth and growth. Plt: platelets. RBC: red blood cells. WBC: white blood cells.

sidered that acceleration of thrombolysis is due to vibration of thrombus, acceleration of tPA diffusion into the thrombus, acceleration of the effects of tPA by increasing tissue temperature, and/or cavitation.[8]

We have observed the effects of ultrasound irradiation on carotid artery thrombus in dogs.[9] With low output, the thrombus vibrated and detachment of blood corpuscles was increased. With higher output,

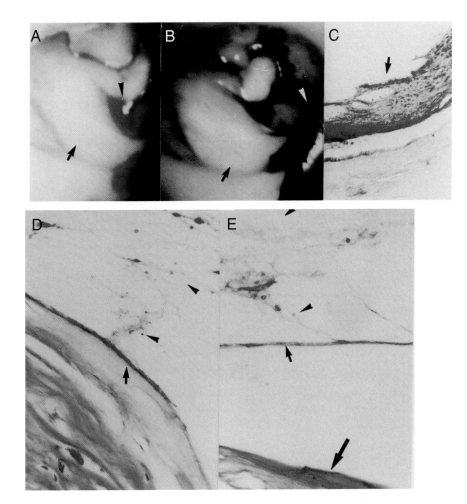

Fig. 10. Isolated human atherosclerotic coronary artery perfused with canine arterial blood. **A:** 10 minutes after blood perfusion. Arrow: ulcer. **B:** after Evans blue. **C:** oil red O stain. Arrowheads in A and B: thrombus. Note: thrombus in the surrounding portions of but not in the ulcer. **D:** fibrin growth from the endothelial cells. **E:** fibrin growth from the exfoliated endothelial cells but not from the collagen fibers beneath. Arrowheads in D and E: fibrin network. Arrow in D and small arrow in E: endothelial cells. Larger arrow in E: collagen fibers.

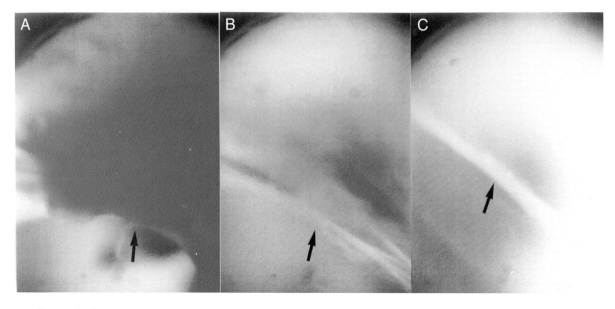

Fig. 11. Effects of saline perfusion on thrombus color. **A:** red thrombus before saline perfusion (arrow). **B:** pink thrombus with white bands 10 minutes after saline infusion (arrow). **C:** white thrombus 30 minutes after saline infusion. Exposed bundle-like structure (arrow).

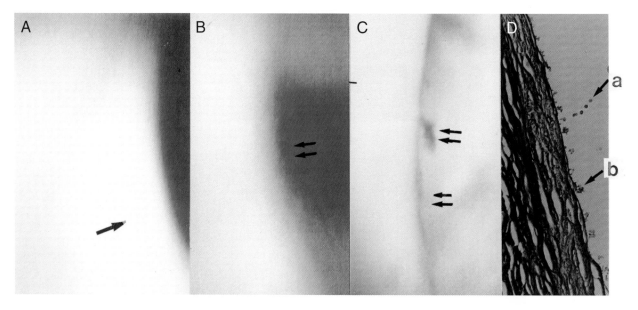

Fig. 12. Isolated human coronary artery. **A:** before blood perfusion. **B:** after saline infusion performed after thrombus formation. Arrows: frosty glass-like surface. **C:** Evans blue stain. Arrows: cotton candy-like blue structures that correspond to **a** and **b** in D. **D:** histological changes of the same artery. **a:** blood corpuscles on fibrin thread. **b:** platelets. Azan stain ×400.

microbubbles appeared from the thrombus (Fig. 15C; Table 3). Histologically, fibrin networks were disrupted with low output and multiple microcavities were formed in the thrombus with high output (Fig. 15D–F).[10] This new therapeutic modality can be clinically used to reduce bleeding.

Thrombosis and Thrombolysis in Coronary Stents

Coronary stents act as the site of thrombus formation, due to flow turbulence and their affinity to fi-

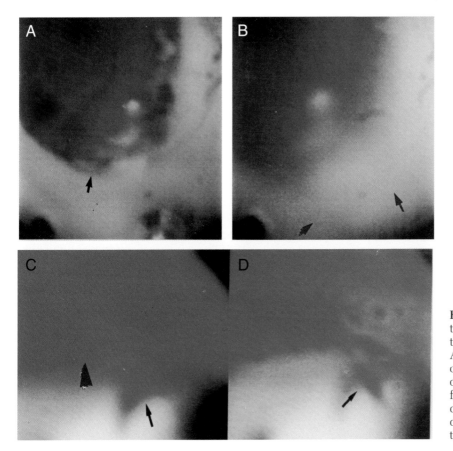

Fig. 13. Thrombolysis of a globular thrombus (30 min in age). **A:** red globular thrombus before. **B:** during tPA infusion. Arrows in B: sandstorm-like dispersion of blood corpuscles. **C** and **D:** detachment of significantly large lumps of thrombus from mother thrombus (10 min in age) during tPA infusion. Arrows: detached daughter thrombi. Arrowhead: mother thrombus.

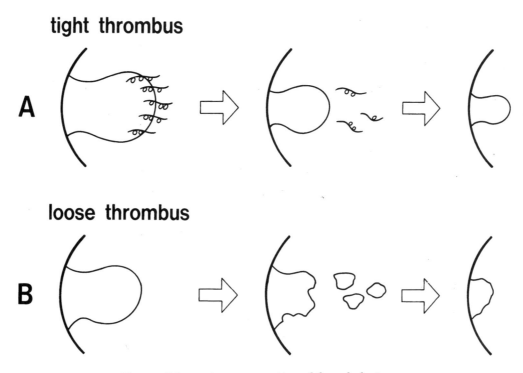

Fig. 14. Schematic representation of thrombolysis.

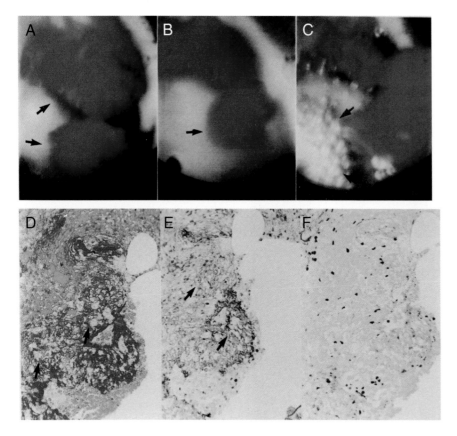

Fig. 15. Effects of ultrasound irradiation through adventitia on arterial thrombus in canine carotid artery. **A:** before irradiation. **B:** ultrasound irradiation combined with tPA infusion. Vibration of thrombus and dispersion of blood corpuscles (arrow). **C:** gas bubbles from the thrombus due to cavitation (arrow) during irradiation. **D:** Azan stain. Multiple cavities in the thrombus. **E:** TPHA stain. Note: disruption and fragmentation of fibrin (arrows). **F:** Giemza stain. Fragmented or vacuolated white blood cells. ×200.

brin and platelets. Protrusion of stent struts into the lumen disturbs laminal flow and accelerates thrombus formation (see section: *Bloodstream in the Stenotic Native Artery*). Immediately after the beginning of blood perfusion through any type of stent, thrombus formation on the stent struts occurs promptly (Fig. 16A–C). It occurs most dominantly at the proximal and distal edges. The color of thrombus is red, white or mixed, or pink. Different from the thrombus at the stenotic segment of native artery, thin cotton candy-like white matter begins to wrap the stent struts immediately after the beginning of blood perfusion. This phenomenon resembles cotton candy formation (Figs. 16D-F). Then, red blood cells are incorporated into them, finally forming a mural or globular red thrombus. However, red blood cells are washed out and bundle or web formation frequently occurs, as in case of saline infusion. They are diffusely stained in blue with Evans blue, indicating that the cotton candy-like matter is mainly composed

Table 3
Effects of Ultrasound Irradiation on Arterial Thrombus During Thrombolytic Therapy With tPA

Output of Ultrasound (KHz,)	100	200	500	1000
1. On aventitia (n = 6)				
Thrombolysis (n = 6)	3	6	6	6
Vibration	2	2	3	5
Cavitation	0	2	4	6
Burn of adventitia	0	0	3	6
2. Transcutaneous (n = 5)*				
Thrombolysis	0	4	5	5
Vibration	0	2	2	3
Cavitation	0	0	1	2
Burn of skin	0	0	2	5

*Distance from skin surface to vessel: 10 mm.

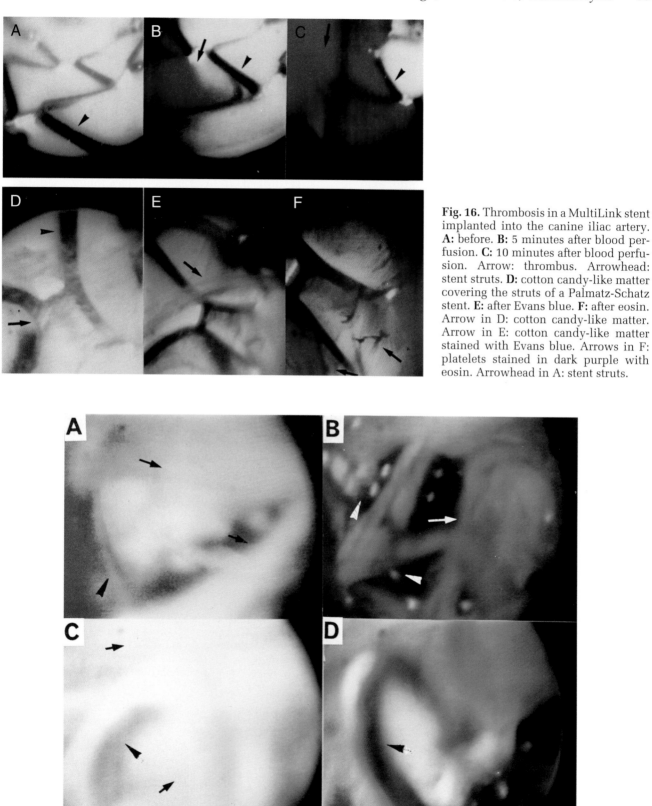

Fig. 16. Thrombosis in a MultiLink stent implanted into the canine iliac artery. **A:** before. **B:** 5 minutes after blood perfusion. **C:** 10 minutes after blood perfusion. Arrow: thrombus. Arrowhead: stent struts. **D:** cotton candy-like matter covering the struts of a Palmatz-Schatz stent. **E:** after Evans blue. **F:** after eosin. Arrow in D: cotton candy-like matter. Arrow in E: cotton candy-like matter stained with Evans blue. Arrows in F: platelets stained in dark purple with eosin. Arrowhead in A: stent struts.

Fig. 17. Magnified angiomicroscopic images of in-stent thrombosis. **A:** web formation at the distal edge of an incompletely expanded stent (arrows). **B:** web was stained with Evans blue, indicating fibrin is its main component. **C:** cotton candy-like matter wrapping the stent struts (arrows). **D:** staining with Evans blue. Arrowheads in A to D: stent struts.

of fibrin. Bundles, webs, and cotton candy-like matter are stained in purple but partially with eosin, indicating that platelets are not playing the major role in their formation.

In case of insufficient expansion of the stent, bundle or web formation often results in complete occlusion (Fig. 17). This fact indicates that complete expansion of the stent so as not to protrude into the lumen is very important for prevention of thrombus-induced acute or subacute in-stent occlusion, a serious complication that is not infrequently experienced in clinical setting.

Since the main component of bundle and web is fibrin, fibrinolytic therapy should be recommended when the same phenomenon is observed by angioscopy during or after stenting. According to our animal experiments, it is difficult to eliminate all of these thrombi with thrombolytic agents. On the other hand, pretreatment with batroxobin, which prevents fi-

brin formation, completely prevented these thrombi.[10] Therefore, use of drugs that prevent fibrin formation, or development of stents that have no affinity to fibrin should be taken into consideration.

Identification of Thrombus by IVUS

Ultrasonographic appearance of thrombus was first described by Natesa.[11] Thrombus exhibits a granulated or nongranulated high echoic mass. However, in the clinical situation, composition and distribution in the same thrombus differ patient to patient. In addition, atheromatous debris of the disrupted plaque is mixed with thrombus. Therefore, the ultrasonographic appearance may differ from thrombus to thrombus. This may be one reason for difficulty of thrombus identification by IVUS.

References

1. Uchida Y, Tomaru T, Kato A, et al: Angioscopy of blood flow through stenotic arteries: Rheologic mechanisms of thrombosis. Am Heart J 114:1504–1506, 1987.
2. Uchida Y, Tomaru T, Sumino S, et al: Fiberoptic observation of thrombosis and thrombolysis in isolated human coronary artery. Am Heart J 112:694–696, 1986.
3. Robbins SL, Bentov I: The kinetics of viscous flow in a model vessel: Effects of stenoses of varying size, shape and length. Lab Invest 16:864–874, 1967.
4. Karini T, Goldsmith HL, Motomiya M: Flow patterns in vessels: Simple and complex geometries. In: Blood in Contact with Natural and Artificial Surfaces. Leonard EF, Turrito WT, Vroman L (eds). Academic Press, NY, 1987, pp 422–441.
5. Chuang PT, Cheng HJ, Lin SJ: Macromolecular transport across arterial and venous endothelium in rats: Studied with Evans blue-albumin and horseradish peroxidase. Arteriosclerosis 10:188–197, 1990.
6. Christensen BC, Chemnitz J, Tkocz I: Repair in arterial tissue: The role of endothelium in the permeability of a healing intimal surface. Vital staining with Evans

blue and silver-staining of the aortic intima after a single dilatation trauma. Act Pathol Microbiol Scand 85:297–310, 1977.
7. Uchida Y, Morita T, Nakamura N: Observation of atherosclerotic lesions by an intravascular microscope in patients with arteriosclerosis obliterance. Am Heart J 130:1114–1119, 1995.
8. Sekiguch H: A new thrombolytic therapy using ultrasound irradiation. J Jikei Med 109:863–871, 1994 (in Japanese).
9. Koga J, Matsuyama A, Sekiguchi H, et al: Angiomicroscopic observation of the effects of ultrasound irradiation on thrombus. Jpn Circulat J 64(Suppl):437, 2000 (in Japanese).
10. Matsuyama A, Koga J, Aoki T, et al: Angiomicroscopic observation of thrombosis and thrombolysis in stent. Proceedings of Jpn Coll Endovasc Interven, p 84, 2000.
11. Natesa G, Andreas K, Brockway B: Detection of intra-arterial thrombus by intravascular high frequency two-dimensional ultrasound imaging in vitro and in vivo studies. Am J Cardiol 65:1280–1283, 1990.

Chapter 10

Clinical Classification of Atherosclerotic Coronary Plaques

Ambrose classified coronary plaques by angiography.[1] His classification is widely used. Fig. 1 shows his classification partly modified by us. The plaques are classified into regular (nondisrupted) and complex (disrupted) plaques. However, the correlation of angioscopic to angiographic classification is still not established.

Plaque Classification by Angioscopy

The histological classification recommended by AHA Council[2] is clinically not fully applicable for plaques by angioscopy and intravascular ultrasound since it is beyond the discrimination power of conventional angioscopes and intravascular ultrasound (IVUS) probes.

Figs. 2–4 show angioscopic appearances of coronary plaques and Table 1 summarizes their characteristics and histological interpretations.

Angioscopically, atherosclerotic masses that protrude into the coronary lumen when observed longitudinally are called coronary plaques. They are classified from surface morphology into regular (smooth and without obvious disruption) (Figs. 2A and 2B) and complex (irregular surface, usually with disruption sometimes accompanied by hemorrhage, hematoma, and thrombus, etc.) (Figs. 3A and 3B).[3–5]

Regular and complex plaques are called "simple plaque" and "complicated plaque" in some of the literature, respectively. The plaques are also classified from surface color into white, light yellow, yellow, brown, white, and yellow in mosaic fashion.[6,7] Based on histological examinations,[8] we classified yellow regular plaques into nonglistening and glistening yellow plaques since the latter category is considered histologically more vulnerable than others (see Chapter 5). The plaques with a frosty glass-like surface or an uneven surface without obvious disruption were included into the complex plaque category.[9] These minimal changes were hardly detectable by angiography and IVUS. The plaques with a smooth surface but accompanied by prestenotic or poststenotic thrombi are also included with complex plaques (Figs. 4A and 4B).[7] Furthermore, regular plaques are classified into nonprotruded (lined) and protruded when observed coaxially, and concentric and eccentric when observed longitudinally (Table 1).

Angioscopic Classification System for Coronary Plaque

The angioscopic classification system for coronary plaque and thrombus was proposed by den Heijer.[10] Table 2 shows his classification partly modified by us.

Relationship Between Angioscopic and IVUS Images

Fig. 5 shows IVUS images of coronary plaques, and Table 3[11] summarizes their characteristics. By IVUS, the coronary plaques are classified, based on their echogenicity when compared to that of adventitia, into hard, soft, mixed, and calcified (Fig. 5A–C). High echogenicity without shadow is generally believed to be due to fibrotic plaques, high echogenicity with shadow due to calcium deposition, and low echogenicity due to atheromatous (lipid-rich) plaques. However, calcium deposition without a shadow behind does exist. Even when the body of plaque is high echoic, the rims are sometimes low echoic (Fig. 5D,E). When both high and low echogenicity exist, the plaque is called mixed. When echogenicity is very low, its ex-

regular plaques   complex plaques

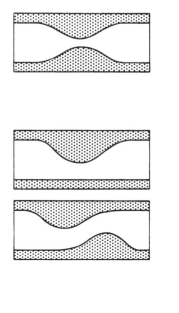

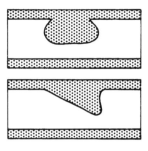

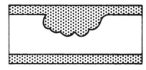

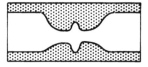

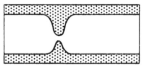

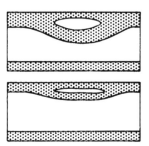

Fig. 1. Modified angiographic classification of coronary plaque. Used with permission from ref. 1.

istence cannot be identified unless positive contrast or negative contrast is injected (Fig. 5F–H). Based on coaxial morphology, the plaques are classified into concentric and eccentric. Based on the presence or absence of a high echoic mass with an echolucent shadow behind, the plaques are classified into those with and without calcium deposition. Based on distribution, calcification is classified as superficial, middle, deep, and disseminated (Fig. 5I–K). [12,13] Figs. 6 and 7 show the relationship between angioscopic and IVUS images of exposed calcium. In Fig. 6, sharp-edged white matter protruded into the lumen. By IVUS, the matter was superficially deposited calcium. In Fig. 7, multiple transparent to white matter was exposed into

the lumen. They reflected illumination. By IVUS, they had shadows behind, indicating that they were calcium crystals, probably ejected from the lipid pool. Histological correlations between angioscopic and IVUS images are shown in Chapter 5.

Although large hemorrhages, ulcers, clefts, dissections, and intimal flaps can be identified (Figs. 8 and 9), they cannot be discriminated by conventional IVUS probes[12–14] when they are less than 50–500 μm in diameter. Presence or absence of a lipid pool inside can be identified only in selected plaques (see Chapter 5). In contrast to angioscopy, conventional IVUS is very weak in identification of fine surface lesions and also in identification of thrombus.

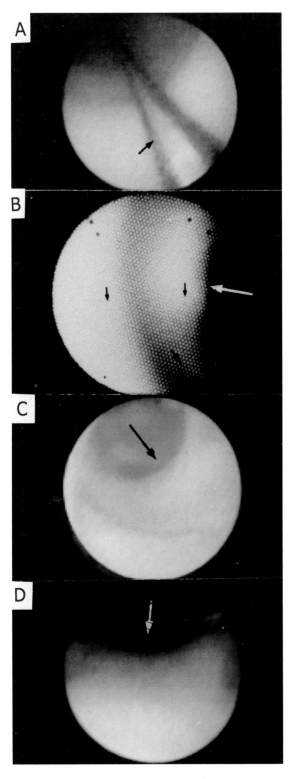

Fig. 2A. Regular coronary plaques. **A:** angiographically normal coronary artery. Smooth and milky white. **B:** white plaque. **C:** light yellow plaque. **D:** nonglistening yellow plaque.

Fig. 2B. Regular coronary plaques. **E:** glistening yellow plaque. **F:** light yellow restenotic plaque after PTCA. **G:** white restenotic plaque after PTCA. **H:** bluish white restenotic plaque after PTCA.

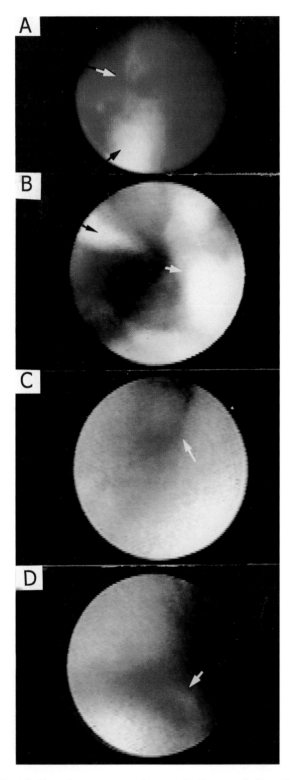

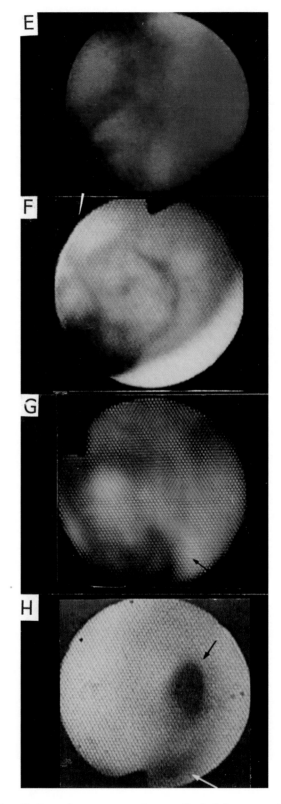

Fig. 3A. Complex coronary plaques. **A:** Fractured glistening yellow plaque (black arrow) covered with occlusive red thrombus (white arrow). **B:** multiple intimal flaps (white arrow) and mural thrombi. Black arrow: guidewire. **C:** a large intimal flap obstructing the lumen (white arrow). **D:** intimal dissection with a small entry (white arrow).

Fig. 3B. Complex coronary plaques. **E:** dark brown and uneven surface with thrombus. **F:** white and brown speckled and uneven surface. **G:** yellowish brown (dirty, resembling feces) and irregular surface. **H:** white and smooth plaque (black arrow) with prestenotic dark red thrombus (white arrow).

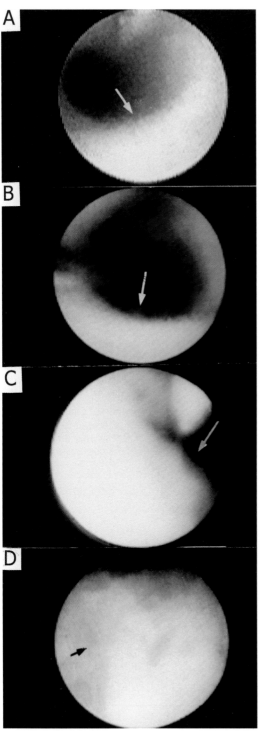

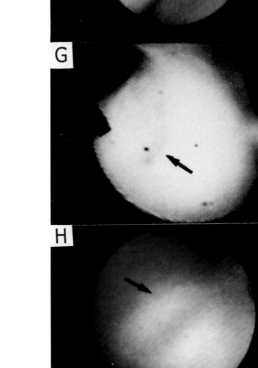

Fig. 4A. Complex plaques that could not be identified by angiography. **A:** white and frosted glass-like surface (injured endothelial cells, fibrin, and platelet aggregates). **B:** yellow and frosted glass-like surface (mixture of fibrin, platelets, injured endothelial cells, and atheromatous substances). **C:** white and uneven surface (endothelial exfoliation. **D:** uneven surface (endothelial exfoliation and subendothelial damage).

Fig. 4B. Complex plaques that could not be identified by angiography. **E:** erosion (white arrows). A shallow hollow with visible irregular margin (exfoliated endothelial cells) and bleeding in the hollow area. **F:** bleeding, purplish, suggesting venous bleeding (arrow). **G:** bleeding, purplish black, suggesting venous bleeding (arrow). Acute coronary syndromes occurred 2 months after angioscopic observation in this patient. **H:** intima with pseudolumen beneath, which was inflated or deflated synchronously with each cardiac beat (arrow).

Table 1
Angioscopic Classification of Coronary Plaques

Classification	*Histopathological Interpretation*	
1. Regular plaque	smooth surface, nondisrupted	
White	fibrous (collagen fiber-rich), no lipid deposition in superficial layer with or without lipid pool	
Light yellow	slight lipid deposition in collagen fiber-rich superficial layer with or without lipid pool; stable	
Nonglistening yellow	abundant lipid deposition in collagen fiber-deficient superficial layer with or without lipid pool; fibrous cap may be thin; relatively vulnerable	
Nonglistening brown	abundant lipid deposition in collagen fiber-reduced superficial layer with or without lipid pool; or organized thrombus; relatively vulnerable	
White and nonglistening yellow in mosaic fashion	sporadic lipid deposition in collagen fiber-rich superficial layer; stable	
Glistening yellow plaque	abundant deposition of lipid, calcium particles, and ceroids in collagen fiber absent very fragile superficial layer or fibrous cap; vulnerable plaque	
2. Complex plaque	irregular surface, with or without the changes below	disruption (fresh or old)
Hemorrhage	red (arterial) or purplish (venous), not protruded, does not disappear by saline flush; bleeding into the lumen may exist	bleeding from vasa vasorum
Hematoma	red or dark red mass seen through, not protruded, does not disappear by saline flush	
Erosion	shallow superficial defect with or without mural thrombus	exfoliation of superficial layer not extended to lipid pool
Ulcer	deep defect with exposed atheromatous tissues; may be covered by a residual fibrous cap or thrombus	residual cavity after gushing forth of lipid pool contents
Cleft or fissuring	longitudinal or coaxial linear separation	
Intimal flap	white or yellow thick flap protruding into the lumen; flutters sometimes; discrimination from thrombus difficult	usually exfoliated fibrous cap
Dissection	swelling of intima on pseudolumen waves sometimes, entry can be detected	separation of intima from media
Fracture	exposed multiple and irregular plaque tissues, usually with multiple intimal flaps and thrombi	complicated disruption of almost entire plaque
3. Unclassified (may be artifact due to procedure)		
Endothelial exfoliation	thin and small white threads with fluttering; difficult to discriminate from fibrin threads	
Frosty glass-like surface	resembles frosted glass, stained with Evans blue	fibrin threads with platelet aggregates on extensively damaged endothelium or erosion; (can be observed in patients with unstable angina)

Table 2
Angioscopic Classification System for Coronary Plaque and Thrombus

Descriptive Items	*Categories*
Image quality	1. adequate
	2. inadequate
Obtained image of target	1. image not recognizable
	2. only vessel wall, lumen not visible
	3. vessel wall, lumen incomplete
	4. vessel wall, complete lumen
	5. central lumen visualization (bull's eye)
Lumen diameter	0. not assessable, not applicable
	1. no or minimal narrowing
	2. narrowing
	3. total occlusion
Shape of narrowing	0. not assessable not applicable
	1. round or elliptical
	2. slit-like
	3 complex shaped
Vessel surface description	0. not assessable, not applicable
	1. smooth
	2. nonmobile protruding irregularities
	3. mobile protruding irregularities
	4. both mobile and nonmobile protruding irregularities
Color of surface	1. homogeneous color
	2. patchy color (mixed, multiple)
white	1. present
bluish white	1. present
light yellow	1. present
nonglistening yellow	1. present
glistening yellow	1. present
brown	1. present
red	1. present
pink	1. present

Diagnostic Items *Categories*	
Plaque	0. not assessable
	1. none
	2. lining
	3. protruding
Disruption	0. not assessable, not applicable
	1. none
	2. small surface disruptions (flaps)
	3. large dissection
	4. large mobile flap(s)
Thrombus	0. not assessable, not applicable
	1. none
	2. amorphous
red, pink, mixed, yellow, brown	3. 1 lining thrombus
	4. multiple lining thrombus
	5. protruding thrombus

Used with permission from ref. 10.

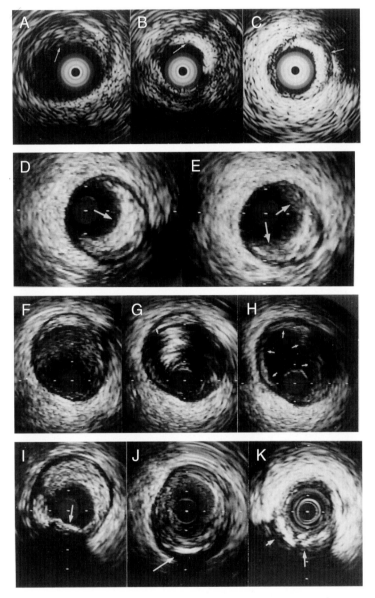

Fig. 5. IVUS images of coronary plaques. **A:** eccentric soft plaque (arrow). **B:** eccentric hard plaque (arrow). **C:** eccentric calcified plaque (arrow). **D:** eccentric hard plaque. **E:** soft rims at the proximal portion of the same plaque as in D. (arrows). **F–H:** Very soft plaque. **F:** before contrast material. **G:** positive contrasting with contrast material with microbubbles. **H:** negative contrasting with saline. The plaque became visible during negative contrasting (arrows). Calcification. **I:** superficial calcification (arrow). **J:** deep calcification (arrow). **K:** disseminated calcification (arrows).

Table 3
Classification of Coronary Plaques by IVUS

1. **Atherosclerotic burden**	Histology
Normal intima	single layer appearance or 3-layer appearance with intimal thickness <0.3 mm
Minimal atherosclerotic burden	<20% of VA occupied by plaque
Moderate atherosclerotic burden	>20% <40% of VA occupied by plaque
Massive atherosclerotic burden	>60% of VA occupied by plaque

2. **Quantitative definitions**

a. *Plaque components*	*Histology*
Echographic characteristics	
Echoreflectivity<than adventitia	fibrocellular tissue, thrombus
Echoreflectivity>than adventitia	dense fibrous tissue
High echoreflectivity + shadowing	calcium

b. *Plaque characteristics*	
homogeneous	*mixed*
soft fibrous	calcific soft/fibrous
low high	high
echoreflective echorefrective	echoreflective soft/calcific
	+shadowing
	fibrocalcific

c. *Wall disruption*	
Rupture	radial tear, perpendicular to the vessel wall
Dissection	longitudinal tear, parallel to the vessel wall
Location	proximal, distal, at target stenosis
Axial length	in mm
Circumferential extension	arch in hours or degrees
Maximum depth partial	plaque between tear and adventitia
complete	full thickness tear extending through the plaque to the adventitia

VA: total vessel area.
Used with permission from ref. 11.

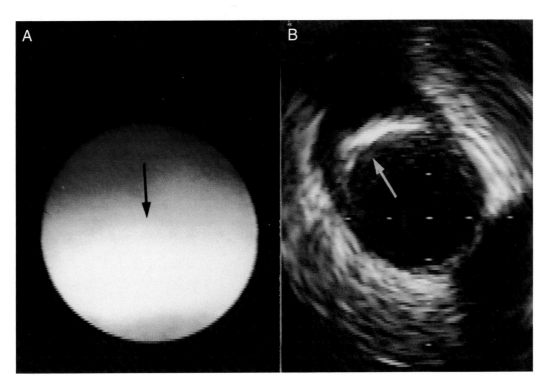

Fig. 6. A: sharp-edged white matter protruding into the lumen (arrow). **B:** IVUS image of the same matter. Shadow behind indicates calcium.

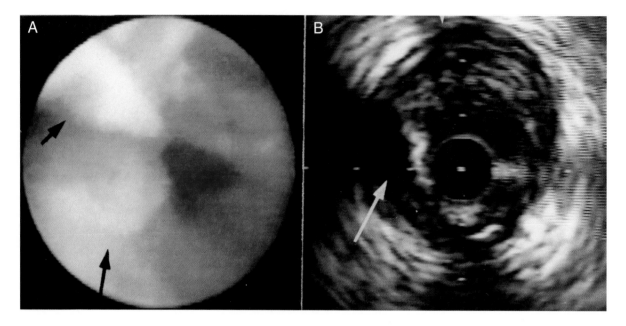

Fig. 7. A: multiple sharp-edged transparent or white matter exposed into the lumen. **B:** IVUS image showing high echogenicity with shadow behind, indicating calcium crystals.

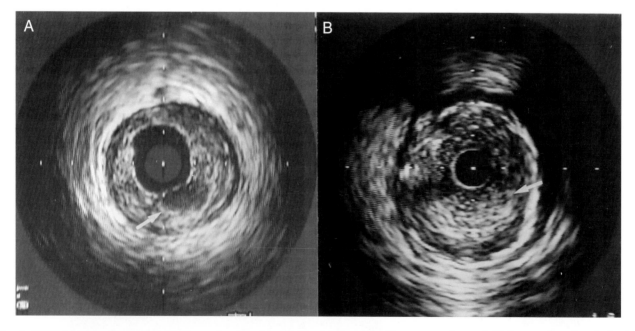

Fig. 8. IVUS images of complex plaques. **A:** ulcer (cavity) beneath a thin fibrous cap (arrow). **B:** Large ulcer (cavity) with high echoic fluid inside (arrow). Both cavities are possibly vacant spaces remaining after ejection of the atheromatous debris and filled with liquid.

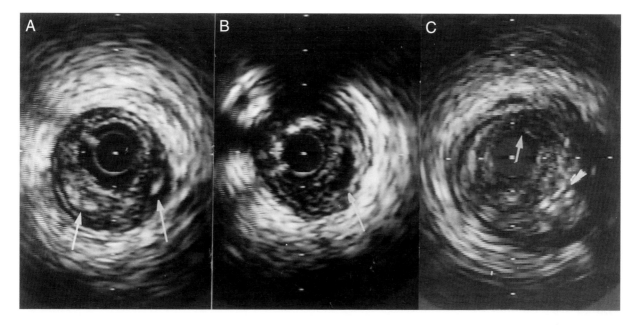

Fig. 9. IVUS images of complex plaques. **A:** mixed plaque with 2 homogeneous high echoic spaces margined by a low echoic space, suggesting hemorrhage (arrows). **B:** soft plaque with a echolucent cavity not communicating with the lumen (arrow). **C:** dissection at the rim of a mixed plaque (arrow).

References

1. Ambrose JA, Winters SL, Stern A, et al: Angiographic morphology and the pathogenesis of unstable angina pectoris. J Am Coll Cardiol 5:609–616, 1985.
2. Stary HC, Chandler B, Dinsmore RE, et al: A definition of advanced types of atherosclerotic lesions and histological classification of atherosclerosis. Circulation 92:1355–1374, 1995.
3. Sherman CT, Litvack F, Grundfest W, et al: Coronary angioscopy in patients with unstable angina pectoris. N Engl J Med 315:913–919, 1986.
4. Uchida Y, Tomaru T, Nakamura F, et al: Percutaneous coronary angioscopy in patients with ischemic heart disease. Am Heart J 114:1069–1075,1989.
5. Uchida Y, Hasegawa K, Kawamura K, et al: Angioscopic observation of coronary changes induced by percutaneous transluminal coronary angioscopy. Am Heart J 117:1153–1155, 1989.
6. Uchida Y: Percutaneous coronary angioscopy. Jpn Heart J 33:271–294, 1992.
7. Uchida, Y, Fujimori Y, Ohsawa H, et al: Angioscopic evaluation of stabilizing effects of bezafibrate on coronary plaques. Coronary 16:293–301, 1999.
8. Uchida Y, Kanai M, Takeuchi K, et al: Angioscopic appearance of vulnerable coronary plaques and its patho-logical correlations. Coronary 16:302–313, 1999 (in Japanese).
9. Uchida Y: Angioscopic detection of vulnerable coronary plaques and prediction of acute coronary syndromes. In: The Vulnerable Atherosclerotic Plaques. Fuster V (ed). Futura Publishing Co, Inc., Armonk, NY, 1999, pp 111–129.
10. den Heijer P, Foley DP, Hillege HL, et al: The Ermenoville classification of observations at coronary angioscopy: Evaluation of intra- and interobserver agreement. Eur Heart J 15:815–822, 1994.
11. Di Mario C: Clinical application and image interpretation in intracoronary ultrasound. Eur Heart J 19:207–229, 1998.
12. Porkin BN, Bartorelli AL, Gessert JM, et al: Coronary artery imaging with intravascular high-frequency ultrasound. Circulation 81:1575–1585, 1990.
13. Pandian NG, Kreis A, Brockway B: Detection of intraarterial thrombus by intravascular high-frequency two-dimensional ultrasound imaging: In vitro and in vivo studies. Am J Cardiol 65:1280–1283, 1990.
14. Friedman M, Van den Bovenkamp GJ: The pathogenesis of a coronary thrombus. Am J Pathol 48:19–44, 1997.

Chapter 11

Clinical Classification of Coronary Thrombus

Classification by Angioscopy

den Heijer proposed "The Ermenonville Classification" of coronary thrombus and disruption (dissection).[1] However, coloration of a given thrombus differs when a different angioscope is used and output of the illumination source is changed, especially in the case of white or yellow thrombus. Also, the color of the neighboring wall is reflected on the thrombus and its color is modified. A specific and sensitive method such as quantitative colorimetric angioscopic analysis,[2] by which composition and age of the thrombus can be discriminated, remains to be established.

Table 1 shows our classification of coronary thrombus and its histological correlations based on the data obtained in animal experiments (see Chapter 9). Angioscopically, a predominantly mural mobile or nonmobile mass, adherent to the vessel surface but clearly a separate structure, is classified as thrombus.

Coronary thrombi are classified based on surface color into red, pink or purple, white, white and red in mosaic fashion, dark red, yellow, and brown. The surface color of thrombus is determined by its composition and age. In case of fresh thrombus, color is also influenced by the presence or absence of blood flow or by interventions. Red indicates existence of abundant red blood cells in loose fibrin networks. Pink or purple indicates a reduced number of red blood cells and abundant fibrin and platelets. White indicates that at least the superficial layer is composed of fibrin and/or platelets. Dark red is probably a red blood cell-rich thrombus aged for a few days. According to our animal experiments, yellow indicates an organized thrombus aged at least 2 weeks. The brown may indicate a mixture of atheromatous debris and thrombus, especially when glistening particles are included in it.

The coronary thrombus is also classified, based on its morphology and localization, as amorphous, mural (lining or nonprotruded), globular (protruded), band or web, and streamer-like. Red amorphous configuration indicates red blood cell stagnation in a very loose fibrin network. White amorphous configuration indicates a loose fibrin network with or without platelets aggregated on it.

White band, web, and membranous configurations indicate residual fibrin after washout or autolysis of the thrombus. Streamer-like configuration indicates flow-dependent growth downstream or upstream (Figs. 1–3, Table 1).

Sizing of Thrombus

den Heijer proposed an angioscopic classification for semiquantitative angioscopic assessment of coronary thrombi.[3] Table 2 shows his classification, which we partly modified because his table did not list thrombi yellow or brown in color.

Dye Image Angioscopy for Discrimination of Thrombus Composition

Vital staining with dyes is useful for discrimination of thrombus composition and vessel wall damage.[4,5] Evans blue is routinely used for discrimination of plaque disruption and thrombus composition in our laboratories.

Fig. 4 shows representative examples of dye image angioscopy of coronary thrombi observed in patients with acute coronary syndromes. The red portion of the thrombus was not stained, and white portions were either stained or not stained. Red blood cells have no affinity for this dye. The reason why the red

Table 1
Angioscopic Classification of Coronary Thrombi

Angioscopic Appearance		Histopathological Interpretation
Color	*Surface morphology*	

1. Thrombus that can be identified by conventional angioscopy predominantly mural, mobile or nonmobile, superficial (mural), or protruding (globular) mass, adherent to the vessel wall at least at one portion, but clearly a separate structure

Fresh red	uniformly fresh red	young, red blood cell-rich thrombus, relatively loose fibrin network
Dark red	uniformly dark red	a few days old red blood-cell rich thrombus, relatively loose fibrin network
Pink	uniformly pink	platelet-rich and red blood cell-reduced thrombus
White	uniformly white, shaggy, cotton candy-like, globular, band-like or web-like	fibrin-rich thrombus if stained in blue with Evans blue; platelet-rich thrombus if not fibrin-rich remnant of autolysed thrombus
Mixed	mixed red and white	regional difference in composition
Yellow	uniformly yellow or mixed with red	organized thrombus with or without fresh thrombus
Brown	uniformly brown or mixed with white	organized thrombus if not stained with Evans blue, or mixture of atheromatous debris and fibrin and/or platelets if stained with Evans blue.
Any color with small glistening particles		mixed with calcium and/or cholesterol crystals from disrupted plaque

2. Difficult to identify by conventional angioscopy but can be identified by dye image angioscopy

Red	amorphous but remains even after saline flush	stagnation of red blood cells in very loose fibrin network
White? or not visible	cotton candy-like stained with Evans blue	very loose fibrin thrombus
Frosted glass-like vessel surface	stained in blue with Evans blue	fibrin threads and platelet aggregates

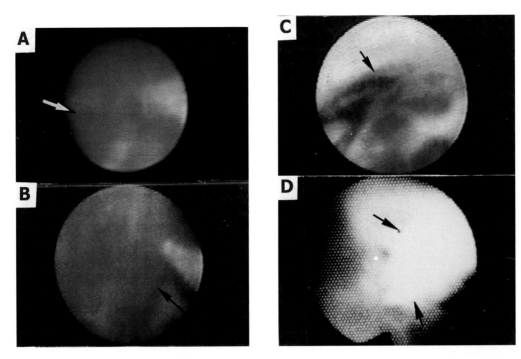

Fig. 1. Commonly observed globular (protruded) coronary thrombi (arrows). **A:** red thrombus. **B:** pink thrombus. **C:** mixed thrombus. **D:** white and cotton candy-like thrombus.

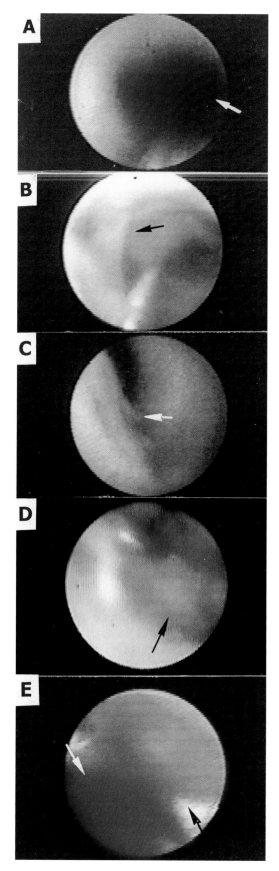

Fig. 2. Less commonly observed thrombi (arrows in each image). **A:** red and amorphous thrombus. **B:** white and membranous thrombus. **C:** white and band thrombus. **D:** brown and cotton candy-like thrombus. **E:** brown and globular mass, probably an organized thrombus or atheromatous debris (black arrow) associated with red and globular thrombus (white arrow).

Angioscopic Classification of Coronary Thrombi

		color	configuration		histology	
A. amorphous thrombi 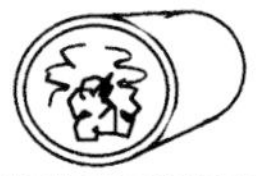		red white	amorphous	loose	loose thrombi loose or tight thrombi	red: RBC rich pink or purple: platelet rich
B. mural thrombi 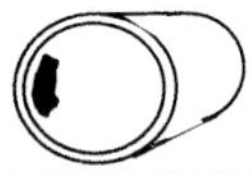		red pink white mixed yellow	patchy doughnut-like	loose tight	thin thrombi	
C. globular thrombi 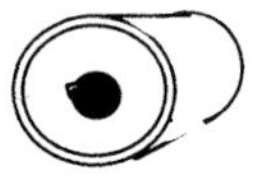		red pink white mixed yellow	globular	loose tight	loose or tight thrombi	white: fibrin rich mixed: non-uniform composition of RBC, platelet and fibrin
D. band thrombi 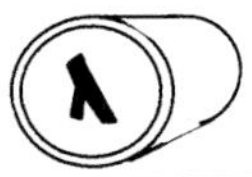		white	bridge-like web-like	 tight	fibrin rich thrombi	
E. streamer-like thrombi 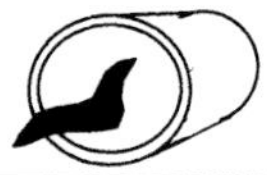		red-tailed pink-tailed purple-tailed white-tailed	streamer-like	loose tight	depends on color	yellow: organized thrombus or lipid brown : lipid
F. B,C		brown			mixed with atheromatous tissue	

Fig. 3. Classification of coronary thrombi based on their configuration.

thrombus was not stained is that its surface was composed mainly of red blood cells. Since fibrin (but not platelets) has affinity for this dye, the white thrombus stained was composed mainly of fibrin and that not stained was composed mainly of platelets. In animal experiments, platelets are stained in purple with a combination of Evans blue and eosin. However, since the clinical safety of eosin has not been proven, staining with eosin was not performed. The exposed interior of the yellow ulcerated portion was not stained as in vitro study (see Chapter 9), indicating that atheromatous tissues have no affinity for Evans blue.

On the other hand, the intimal flaps around the ulcer were stained in the majority of plaques, indicating that the endothelial cells on the flaps had been damaged (Table 3).[6]

Modification of Thrombus by Saline Flush and Guidewire Passing

Fig. 5 shows the effects of repeated saline flush on a mural thrombus in a patient with acute myo-cardial infarction. The thrombus was pink at the first observation. By repeating saline flush, the color of the thrombus was changed into light pink and finally into white. In our animal experiments, it was revealed that saline flush causes dispersion of red blood cells, resulting in fibrin- and platelet-rich white thrombus. Similar changes are also caused by infusion of thrombolytic agents (see Chapter 9). Also, passing a guidewire through the thrombus results in deformation and fragmentation of the thrombus. For example, a smooth-surfaced tight and white thrombus becomes cotton candy-like by repeated guidewire passing.

Comparison Between Angioscopy and Angiography for Discrimination of Plaque Disruption and Thrombus

Sherman et al. were the first to compare angioscopic and angiographic capability for detection of

Table 2
Modified Angioscopic Classification for Disruption (Dissection), Thrombus and Bleeding

1. Normal vessel
   Vessel wall appearing uniformly smooth in contour, and of a uniform milky white or white. There are no abrupt changes in diameter. The lumen is free of intraluminal structures.

2. Plaque
   a) Regular plaque
      0 Not assessable, not applicable
      1 None. Smooth-surfaced or shallow spiral grooves.
      2 Lining plaque. Nonelevated yellow or white discoloration
      3 Protruding plaque. Nonmobile, elevated and/or protruding yellow, brown or white discoloration. There may be focal or diffuse narrowing.
   b) Complex plaque (disruption)
      0 Not assessable, not applicable.
      1 None
      2 Small surface disruptions.
         Irregular surface
         Frosty surface
         Erosion: small and shallow dent with irregular margins
         Flaps: small, very mobile structures which are contiguous with the vessel wall. They don't impede visualization of the lumen (requires differentiation from fibrin threads and platelet aggregates).
      3 Large surface disruptions. Visible cracks or fissures on the luminal surface and/or large mobile or nonmobile protruding structures, which are contiguous with the vessel wall and of homogeneous appearance with the vessel wall. They impede visualization of the lumen.

3. Thrombus
   Lining thrombus. Predominantly mural, nonmobile, superficial mass, adherent to the vessel surface, but clearly a separate structure. Protruding thrombus. Intraluminal, protruding, mobile or nonmobile mass, adherent to the vessel surface, but clearly a separate structure.
   a) Red thrombus
      0 Not assessable, not applicable
      1 None
      2 One lining thrombus
      3 Multiple lining thrombus
      4 Amorphous thrombus
      5 Protruding thrombus <1/3 of lumen
      6 Protruding thrombus 1/3–2/3 of lumen
      7 Protruding thrombus 2/3–3/3 of lumen
   b) White thrombus
      0 Not assessable, not applicable
      1 None
      2 One lining thrombus
      3 Multiple lining thrombus
      4 Amorphous or cotton candy-like
      5 Protruding thrombus <1/3 of lumen
      6 Protruding thrombus 1/3–2/3 of lumen
      7 Protruding thrombus 1/3–3/3 of lumen
   c) Mixed red/white thrombus
      0 Not assessable, not applicable
      1 None
      2 One lining thrombus
      3 Multiple lining thrombus
      4 Amorphous
      5 Protruding thrombus <1/3 of lumen
      6 Protruding thrombus 1/3–2/3 of lumen
      7 Protruding thrombus 2/3–3/3 of lumen
   d) Yellow thrombus
      0 Not assessable, not applicable
      1 None
      2 One lining thrombus
      3 Multiple lining thrombus
      4 Amorphous, cotton candy-like thrombus
      5 Protruding thrombus <1/3 of lumen

continued

Table 2
Modified Angioscopic Classification for Disruption (Dissection), Thrombus and Bleeding (*continued*)

- 6 Protruding thrombus 1/3–2/3 of lumen
- 7 Protruding thrombus 2/3–3/3 of lumen
- e) Brown thrombus
  - 0 Not assessable, not applicable
  - 1 None
  - 2 One lining thrombus
  - 3 Multiple lining thrombus
  - 4 Amorphous, cotton candy-like
  - 5 Protruding thrombus <1/3 of lumen
  - 6 Protruding thrombus 1/3–2/3 of lumen
  - 7 Protruding thrombus 2/3–3/3 of lumen
- f) Glistening particles in the thrombus
  - 0 No
  - 1 Yes
- g) Evans blue dye
  - 0 Not stained
  - 1 Stained
- h) Visible after Evans blue dye
  - 0 Not assessable, not applicable
  - 1 None
  - 2 One lining thrombus
  - 3 Multiple lining thrombus
  - 4 Amorphous, cotton candy-like
  - 5 Protruded thrombus <1/3
  - 6 Protruded thrombus 1/3–2/3
  - 7 Protruded thrombus 2/3–3/3 of lumen
- i) Length
  - 0 Not assessable, not applicable
  - 1 Short (within one segment)
  - 2 Long (streamer-like, over one segment)
- 4. Hemorrhage
  - 0 Not assessable, not applicable
  - 1 None
  - 2 Present. A distinct, demarcated, red or purple, nonelevated discoloration, which is clearly within the vessel wall.

Used with permission from refs. 1 and 2, and partly modified.

plaque disruption and thrombus. They compared angioscopic findings obtained during open heart surgery with those of preoperative angiography in patients with unstable angina and noticed that angioscopy is superior to angiography in detecting plaque disruption and thrombus.[7] The same results were obtained by the author,[8] Ramee,[9] and others (Table 4).

Comparison Between Angioscopy and IVUS for Discrimination of Plaque Disruption and Thrombus

Bocksch defined a pulsatile low echoic mass on the plaque as thrombus.[10] Chemarin-Alibelli defined a granulated or dotted mass moving synchronously to the flow as thrombus.[11] de Feyter observed low echoic and mixed masses almost equally in angioscopically confirmed thrombus and nonthrombotic plaques.[12] Thus, it is generally believed that conventional IVUS is not feasible for identification of coronary thrombus. Low echoic thrombus is very difficult to discriminate from lipids since they have similar echogenicity.[13] Mixing of thrombus with atheromatous debris also modifies discrimination by IVUS.

Ultrasonographically, obvious intimal tear, flap, discontinuity of intima, and connection between lumen and low echoic space in the plaque are all considered plaque disruption. However, detection of disruption is around 10%, probably due to mixing of thrombus with atheromatous tissue and low discrimination power of the conventional IVUS.[14]

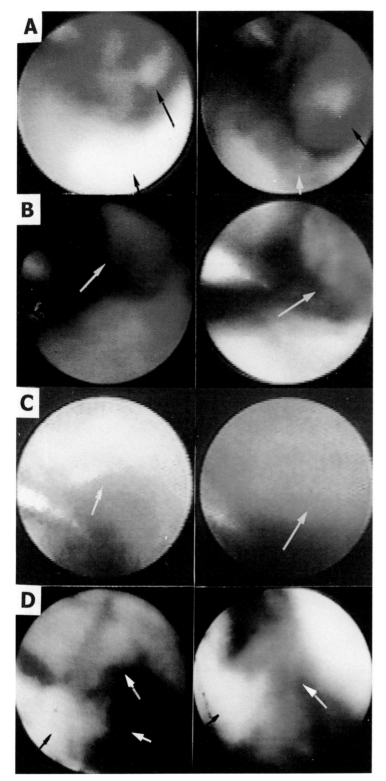

Fig. 4. Dye image angioscopy with Evans blue for discrimination of thrombus composition. **Left:** before staining. **Right:** after staining. **A:** neighboring portions of the red thrombus was stained in blue, indicating a loose fibrin network that was not visible before. **B:** brown and cotton candy-like mass was stained in blue, indicating a mixture of fibrin and atheromatous debris. **C:** light yellow and rough surface was stained in blue, indicating mural fibrin. **D:** white and cotton candy-like thrombus was partially stained and a portion where nothing was observed was also stained, indicating that these portions were fibrin (white arrow) and those not were platelets (black arrow).

Table 3
Dye Staining Angioscopy of Disrupted Coronary Plaques in Patients with Acute Coronary Syndromes (Acute Myocardial Infarction)

	Thrombus			*Flaps*	*Ulcer*
	red	mixed	white		
Stained			1	10	
Not stained	8	4		2	6
Partially stained					1

Wall Hemorrhage

Hemorrhage is also observed in the wall apparently intact by angiography and IVUS. It is usually clearly demarcated, not protruding, and does not disappear by saline flush. It is either red or purple, indicating arterial or venous bleeding, respectively. In the disrupted plaques, bleeding from the wall into the lumen can also be observed. These plaques are either red or purple (Fig. 6).

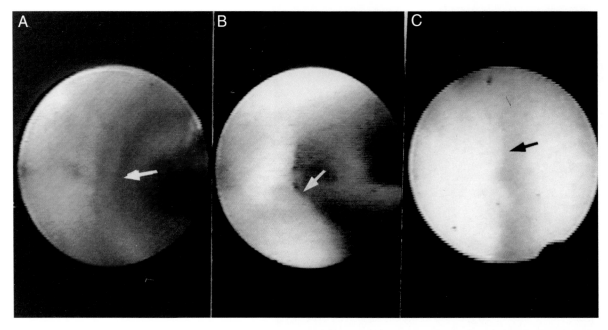

Fig. 5. Changes in thrombus color by repeated saline flush. **A:** pink before saline flush. **B:** almost white after several times of flush. **C:** white after repeated flush.

Table 4
Comparison of Angioscopy and Angiography for Discrimination of Plaque Disruption and Thrombus

	Thrombus		*Disruption*		
	Angioscopy	*CAG*	*Angioscopy*	*CAG*	*Disease*
Sherman CT (1986)	7/10	1/10	4/10	1/10	unstable angina
Uchida Y (1992)	7/26	0/26	13/26	3/26	PTCA
Ramee SR (1991)	2/16	1/16	7/16	0/16	unstable angina
den Heijer P (1994)	31/52	6/52	40/52	15/52	PTCA
Total	19/104	8/104	62/104	19/104	
(%)	18.2	7.6	59.6	18.2	

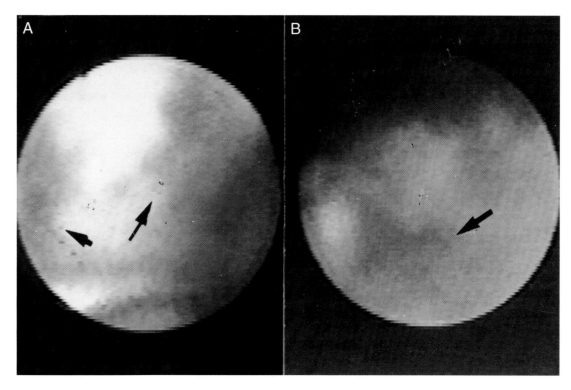

Fig. 6. Wall hemorrhage and bleeding into the lumen. **A:** red, indicating arterial hemorrhage. **B:** purple, indicating venous hemorrhage.

References

1. den Heijer P, Foley DP, Hillege HL, et al: The Ermenonville classification of observations at coronary angioscopy: Evaluation of intra- and interobserver agreement. Eur Heart J 15:815–822, 1994.
2. Lehmann KG, van Suylen RJ, Stibbe J, et al: Composition of human thrombus assessed by quantitative colorimetric angioscopic analysis. Circulation 96:3030–3041, 1997.
3. den Heijer P, Foley DP, Escaned J, et al: Angioscopic versus angiographic detection of intimal dissection and intracoronary thrombus. J Am Coll Cardiol 24:649–654, 1994.
4. Uchida Y, Nakamura F, Morita T: Observation of atherosclerotic plaques by an intravascular microscope in patients with arteriosclerosis obliterance. Am Heart J 130:1114–1117, 1995.
5. Terasawa K, Fujimori Y, Morio H, et al: Evaluation of coronary endothelial cell damages caused by guidewire by in vivo dye staining angioscopy. J Jpn Coll Angiol 40:159–164, 2000.
6. Fujimori Y, Morio H, Terasawa K, et al: Angioscopic evaluation of coronary endothelial lesions by staining with Evans blue in patients with acute myocardial infarction. J Am Coll Cardiol 33(Suppl A):67A, 1999.
7. Sherman T, Litvack F, Grundfest W, et al: Coronary angioscopy in patients with unstable angina pectoris. N Engl J Med 315:913–919, 1986.
8. Uchida Y: Percutaneous coronary angioscopy. Jpn Heart J 33:271–284, 1992.
9. Ramee SR, White JC, Collins TI, et al: Percutaneous angioscopy during coronary angioplasty using a steerable microangioscope. J Am Coll Cardiol 17:100–105, 1991.
10. Bocksch WG, Schartl M, Beckmann S: Intravascular ultrasound in patients with acute myocardial infarction. Eur Heart J 16(Suppl):46–52, 1995.
11. Chemarin-Alibelli MJ, Pieraggi MT, Elbaz M: Identification of coronary thrombus after myocardial infarction by intracoronary ultrasound compared with histology of tissues sampled by atherectomy. Am J Cardiol 77:344–349, 1996.
12. de Feyter PJ, Ozaki Y, Baptista J, et al: Ischemia-related lesion characteristics in patients with stable or unstable angina. Circulation 92:1408–1413, 1995.
13. Jain A, Ramee SR, Mesa J: Intracoronary thrombus: Chronic urokinase perfusion and evaluation with intravascular ultrasound. Cathet Cardiovasc Diagn 26:212–214, 1992.
14. Kawagoe T, Sato M, Tateishi H: Intravascular ultrasound for acute myocardial infarction. In: Cardiovascular Imaging. Igakusyoin Co., Tokyo, 1996, pp 86–94 (in Japanese).

Chapter 12

Relationships Between Angioscopic and Angiographic Images of Coronary Plaques in Different Coronary Syndromes

Coronary artery disease is classified into angina pectoris and acute myocardial infarction. The former is further classified into stable and unstable angina pectoris and the latter into acute and old. Recent coronary imaging revealed that there are keen relationships between plaque morphology and clinical manifestations.

Unstable angina pectoris and acute myocardial infarction have been considered as a consecutive disease process. The concept of unstable angina has emerged from well-known observations that increased frequency and intensity of symptoms were foreboding of the occurrence of acute myocardial infarction. Recent pathological and angioscopic studies revealed that plaque disruption and subsequent local thrombosis were the main clue events in the majority of patients with these disorders, resulting in various degrees of coronary flow reduction and resultant myocardial damages. Therefore, these disorders have been classified as acute coronary syndromes that present a continuum of the disease process and were usually characterized by an abrupt coronary flow reduction[1] (see Chapter 8). Recent angioscopic and pathologic studies, however, revealed some differences between unstable angina and acute myocardial infarction.

Figs. 1–4 show angioscopic images of culprit coronary plaques in different coronary syndromes.[2–11] In stable angina pectoris, the majority of culprit plaques are regular (nondisrupted) plaques with a few exceptions (Fig. 1). The surface color is white in 40–65% of plaques (Fig. 2). Thrombi are observed in a small number of patients with this syndrome (Fig. 3). It is likely that silent disruption occurs in culprit plaques with significant stenosis (see Chapter 8).

In unstable angina pectoris, complex plaques are observed in 30–70% (Fig. 1). The surface color is yellow in 50–85% and thrombus is observed in 25–90%. Why severe ischemic attacks occur in patients with apparently regular plaque and in those without any atherosclerotic plaque remains to be clarified.

In acute myocardial infarction, the majority of plaques are complex, yellow-surfaced, and are associated with thrombus. However, there are a small number of patients in whom thrombus is not detectable (Fig. 3). In old myocardial infarctions, that is, more than 1 month after the onset of the attack, the culprit plaques are complex in 40–75% and thrombi are observed in 35–60% (Fig. 4).

Normal Coronary Artery in Patients with Chest Pain Syndrome

Fig. 5A shows angiographically normal left main trunk (LMT), that is, smooth-surfaced and no obvious stenosis. Angioscopically, the luminal surface was white and smooth (Fig. 5B). Fig. 6A also shows angiographically normal LMT. Angioscopy revealed a smooth yellow luminal surface, indicating lipid deposition in the wall, namely, a fatty streak (Fig. 6B).

Stable Angina Pectoris

Representative Plaques in Stable Angina Pectoris

As mentioned above, the culprit plaques are regular plaques in the majority of patients with stable angina pectoris. Fig. 7 shows a white concentric plaque

93

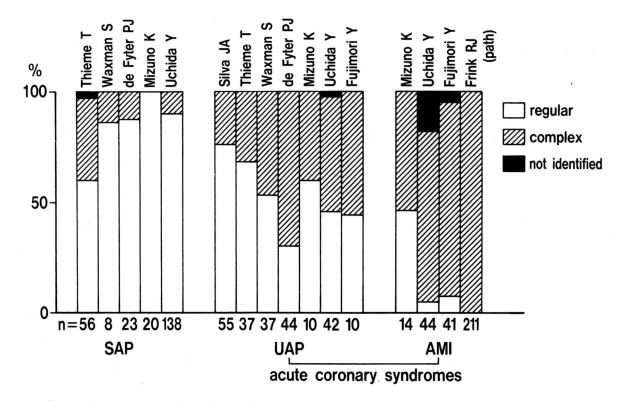

Fig. 1. Incidence of angioscopic regular and complex coronary plaques in different coronary syndromes. SAP: stable angina pectoris. UAP: unstable angina pectoris. AMI: acute myocardial infarction.

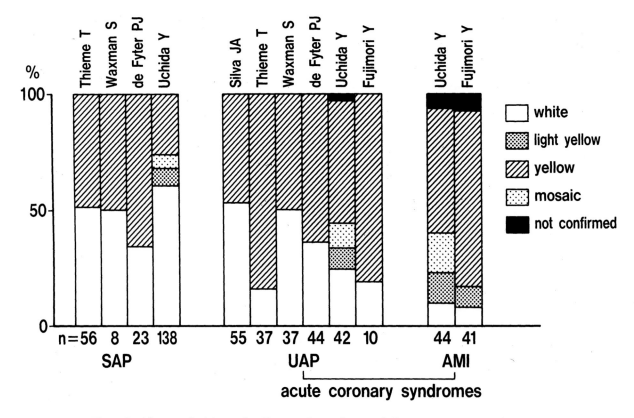

Fig. 2. Incidence of white and yellow surface colors in different coronary syndromes.

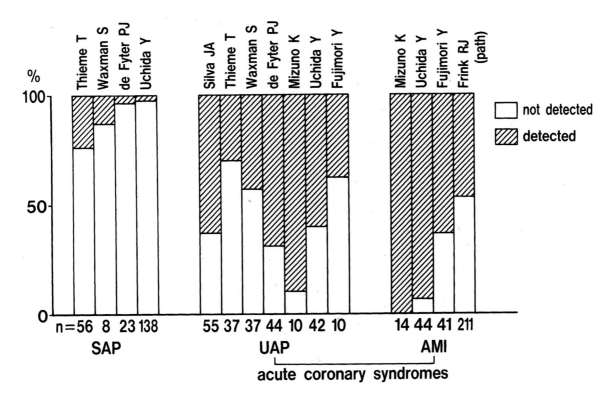

Fig. 3. Incidence of thrombus in different coronary syndromes.

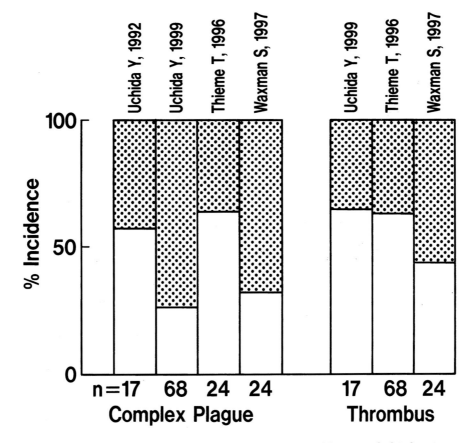

Fig. 4. Incidence of complex plaque and thrombus in old myocardial infarction.

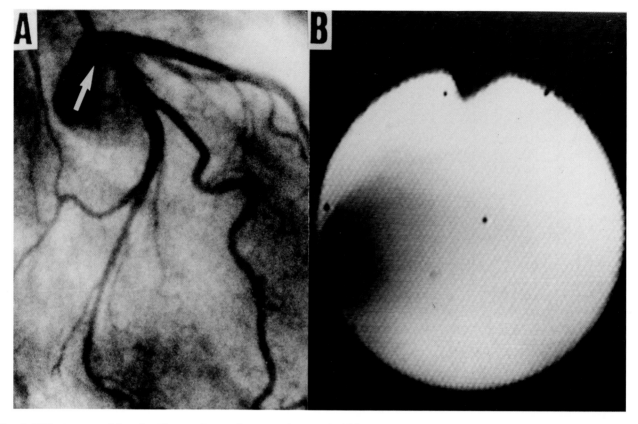

Fig. 5. T.Y., 61-year-old male. Chest pain syndrome without inducible spasm. **A:** angiogram of left coronary artery. Arrow: LMT without plaque. **B:** white and smooth-surfaced LMT.

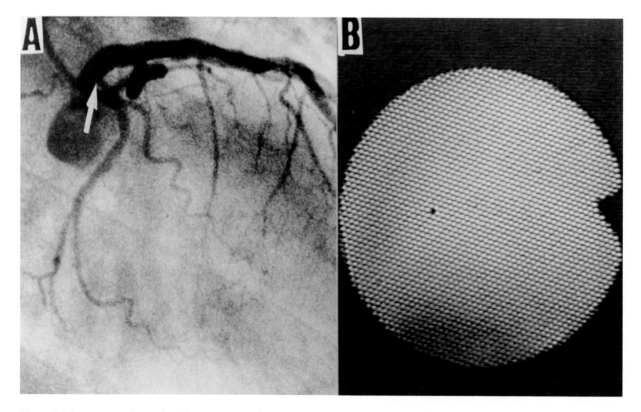

Fig. 6. I.M., 57-year-old male. Chest pain syndrome. **A:** LMT without plaque (arrow). **B:** Yellow and smooth LMT.

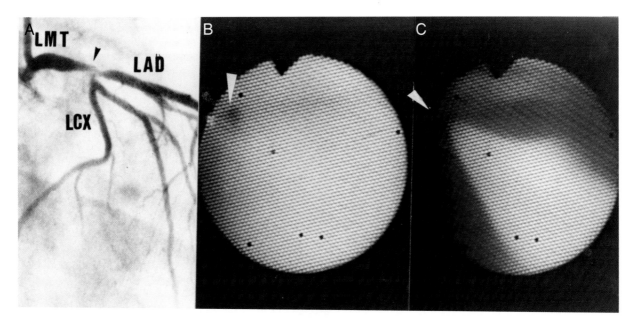

Fig. 7. M.M., 59-year-old male. Stable angina pectoris. **A:** angiogram showing 90% stenosis at the distal end of the LMT involving both the LAD and the LCx. **B:** white and concentric regular plaque occupying the stenotic portion. **C:** bloodstream into the pinhole residual lumen during diastole. Arrowheads in B and C: pinhole residual lumen.

in the distal portion of the LMT. Blood drained into the pinhole residual lumen during diastole. White regular plaques are either concentric or eccentric.

Fig. 8 shows a nonglistening yellow regular plaque observed in the middle segment of the left anterior descending artery (LAD). The plaque was eccentric by both angiography and angioscopy.

Fig. 9 shows a brown regular plaque. The plaque was almost concentric by both angioscopy and angiography.

Fig. 10 shows a glistening yellow plaque in the middle segment of the LAD just distal to the second diagonal branch. In this plaque, the glistening portion was confined to the proximal rim. In our study,

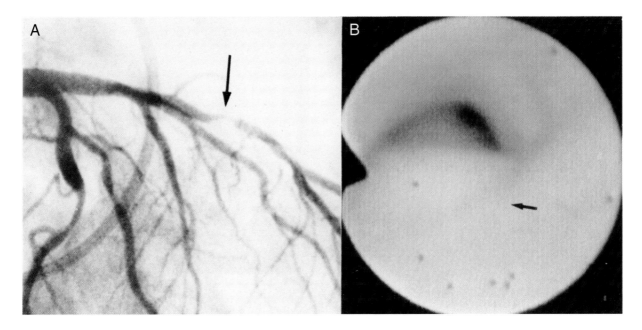

Fig. 8. A.T., 66-year-old female. Stable angina pectoris. **A:** an eccentric and smooth stenosis in the middle segment of the LAD (arrow). **B:** nonglistening yellow and eccentric regular plaque (arrow).

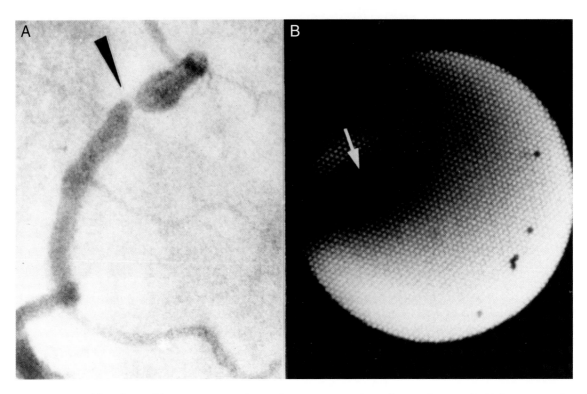

Fig. 9. K.Y., 70-year-old male. Stable angina pectoris. **A:** almost concentric and smooth stenosis. **B:** brown regular plaque.

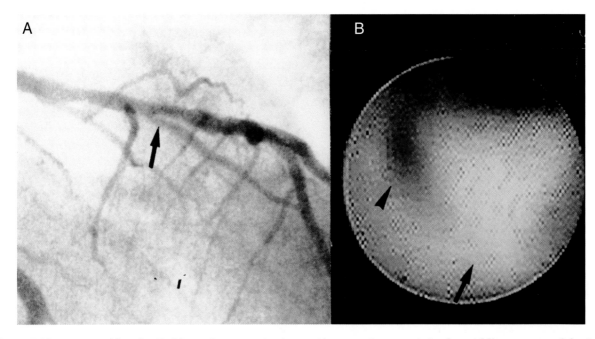

Fig. 10. M.I., 61-year-old male. Stable angina pectoris. **A:** a 25% eccentric stenosis in the middle segment of the LAD, just distal to the second diagonal branch (arrow). **B:** glistening yellow rim of the plaque (arrow) just distal to the ostium of the branch (arrowhead).

glistening yellow plaques were observed in about 5% of regular plaques (Fig. 11).[12]

Multiple Plaques in the Same Coronary Artery

Existence of more than 1 plaque in 1 coronary artery is not infrequent and they often exhibit different images. Fig. 12 shows a glistening yellow plaque in the intermediate branch. This branch had 2 plaques showing narrowings of different severity. In contrast to the glistening yellow plaque in the first stenosis (Fig. 12B), the plaque in the second stenosis (Fig. 12D) was a nonglistening yellow plaque.

Rare Plaques

Fig. 13A shows a slit-like stenosis in the distal segment of the right coronary artery (RCA). The stenosis was due to a membranous plaque (Fig. 13B). Such a membranous plaque was observed in only 2 of 138 plaques in patients with stable angina pectoris. Such a plaque is also observed in the peripheral arteries. However, it is not known whether it is a true atherosclerotic plaque or an organized remnant of fibrin thrombus.

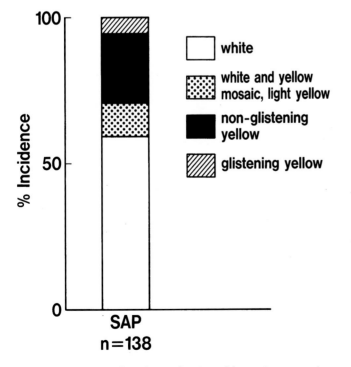

Fig. 11. Incidence of surface color in stable angina pectoris.

Acute Coronary Syndromes

Extensive postmortem microscopic examinations of epicardial coronary arteries in acute coronary syndromes reveal that the majority of thrombi have a layered structure with thrombotic material of differing age, indicating that they were formed successively by repeated mural deposits that caused progressive luminal narrowing over an extended period of time. This episodic growth is accompanied by intermittent fragmentation of thrombus, with peripheral embolization causing microembolic occlusion of small intramyocardial arteries associated with microinfarcts.

Histopathologically, the period of unstable angina before the final attack is characterized by such an ongoing thrombotic process in a major coronary artery where recurrent mural thrombus formation seemed to have alternated with intermittent thrombus fragmentation.[13] Such a dynamic thrombotic process on damaged arteries can easily be reproduced in animal arteries by constriction.[14,15] In our laboratories, coronary angioscopy has been focused on whether or not the same processes actually occur in patients with unstable angina.

Unstable Angina Pectoris

Angioscopically, a variety of luminal changes is observed in the coronary arteries in patients with unstable angina pectoris. Fig. 14 shows angiographic and angioscopic images of the culprit lesion in a patient with unstable angina pectoris. Angiographically, total but hazy obstruction was observed in the middle segment of the LAD. Angioscopically, the hazy obstruction was due to white and cotton candy-like thrombus. By intravascular ultrasound (IVUS), disruption and a small cavity were observed in a segment just proximal to the most stenotic portion. In addition, clefts were observed in the mixed plaque composing the most stenotic portion (Fig. 15).

Fig. 16 shows a coronary angiogram in a patient with unstable angina pectoris. The artery had a 90% stenosis in the middle segment of the LAD. Angioscopy revealed a red thrombus occupying the stenotic portion. Five minutes after the beginning of percutaneous transluminal coronary recanalization (PTCR) with tPA, the thrombus was detached, causing distal embolism and exposing an erosion that had been hidden with the thrombus. The surrounding portions were stained with Evans blue, indicating en-

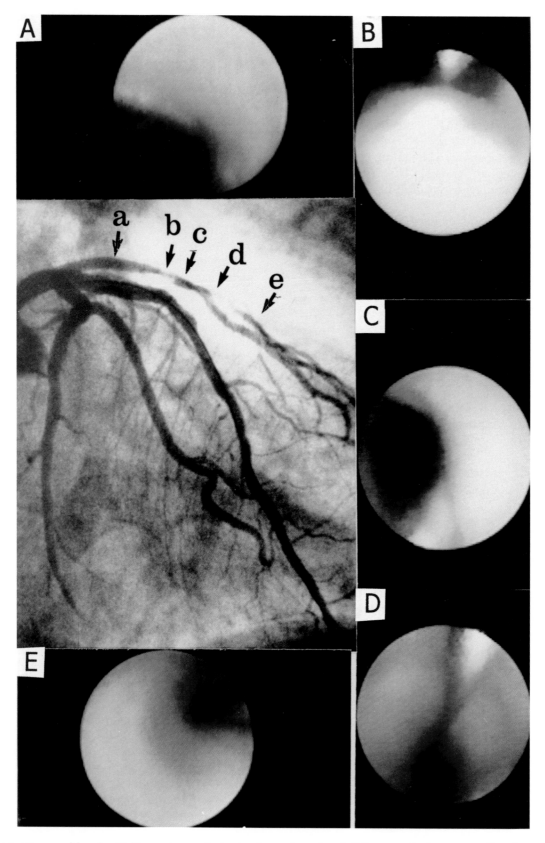

Fig. 12. U.H., 70-year-old male. Stable angina pectoris. Angioscopic regional differences in the intermediate branch. Arrows labeled with **A–E** in the angiogram correspond to those in angioscopic images, respectively.

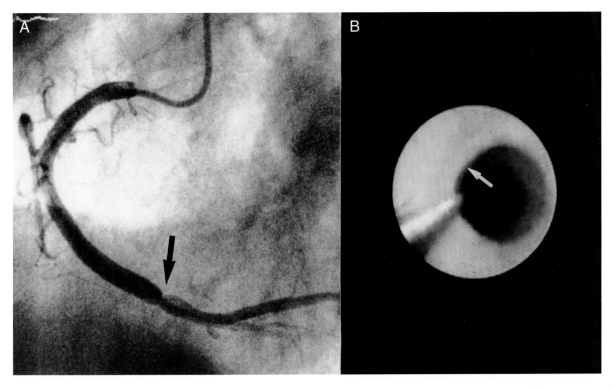

Fig. 13. M.M., 73-year-old female. Stable angina pectoris. **A:** slit-like stenosis in the distal segment of the RCA (arrow). **B:** light yellow concentric and membranous plaque (arrow).

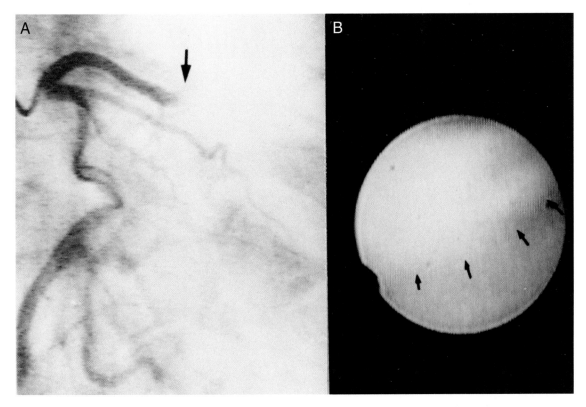

Fig. 14. I.I., 51-year-old male. Unstable angina pectoris. **A:** hazy obstruction in the middle segment of the LAD (arrow). **B:** white and cotton candy-like thrombus (arrows).

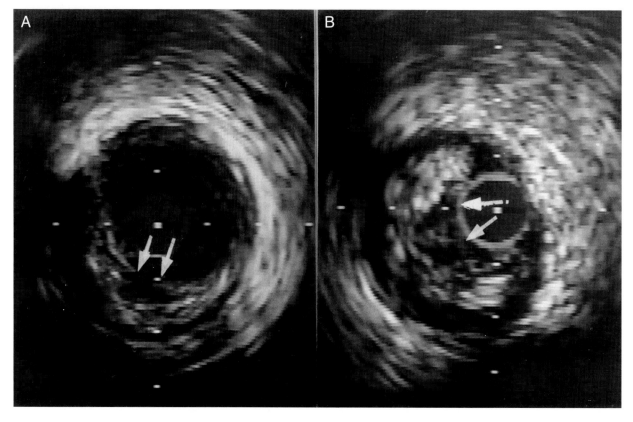

Fig. 15. The same patient as in Fig. 14. **A:** just proximal to the most stenotic portion. Arrows: splitting of intima (arrows) and a cavity beneath. **B:** clefts in the plaque composing the most stenotic portion (arrows).

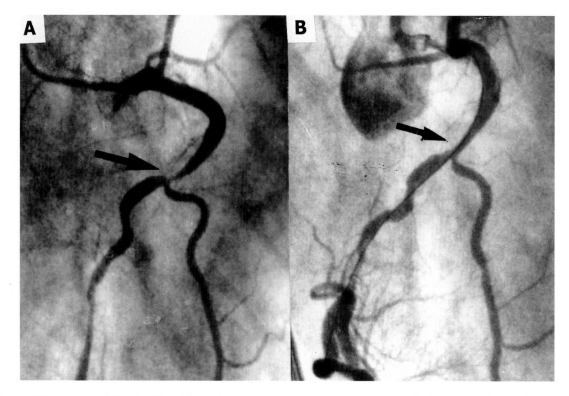

Fig. 16. F.J., 53-year-old male. Unstable angina pectoris. Angiograms of the LAD before (**A**) and after (**B**) PTCR.

dothelial damage and/or remnant fibrin (see Chapter 9) (Fig. 17). Farb reported that superficial erosion of plaques lacking a lipid core was found in 44% of cases of sudden death.[16] Our findings support the concept of Falk that superficial erosion plays an important role in unstable angina pectoris.[13]

Fig. 18 shows an irregular stenosis in the LAD in a patient with unstable angina. Angioscopically, a large flap occupying the lumen was identified. The flap had a red thrombus behind. Probably, the flap obstructed the lumen intermittently, causing periodic anginal attacks. This patient was successfully treated by stent implantation.

In a patient with this syndrome, the middle segment of the left circumflex coronary artery (LCx) was stenotic. Angioscopically, a streamer-like dark red thrombus was observed just proximal to the most stenotic portion (Fig. 19). The thrombus may be formed a few days before and repetitive formation of new thrombus on this thrombus or obstruction of the most stenotic portion with the tail of this thrombus may have induced recurrent anginal attacks.

In about 50% of patients with this category of syndrome, the plaques that were considered culprit for the attack were apparently intact by angiography and also by conventional angioscopy. We noticed that the culprit plaque and its surrounding portions exhibited a frosted glass-like surface in 8 of 11 plaques. To gain insight into the mechanism for this phenomenon, we carried out dye image angioscopy with Evans blue.

Fig. 20 shows angiograms of the LAD in a patient with unstable angina. It was revealed that the middle segment of the LAD had an insignificant stenosis. We performed angioscopy of this segment without the use of a guidewire. The insignificantly stenotic segment exhibited a frosted glass-like luminal surface and it was diffusely stained in blue with Evans blue (Fig. 21). A frosted glass-like surface was observed not only in yellow but also in white plaques and less extensive or focal stain was observed in other patients (Fig. 22).

In our animal experiments, the luminal surface of an artery after washout of the thrombus exhibited

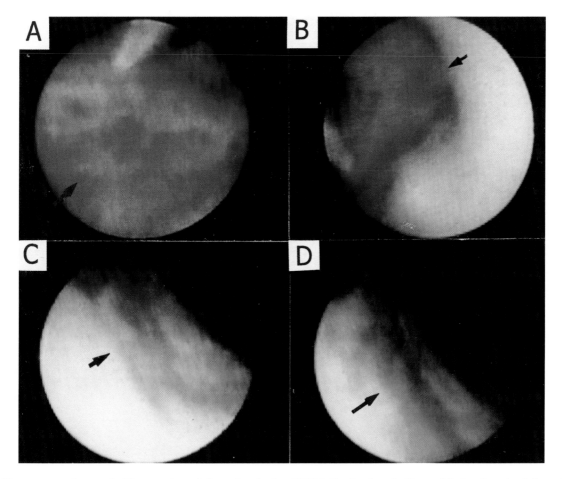

Fig. 17. The same patient as in Fig. 16. **A:** red thrombus before PTCR. **B:** distal embolism with the detached thrombus during PTCR (arrow). **C:** exposed erosion after PTCR (arrow). **D:** after staining with Evans blue.

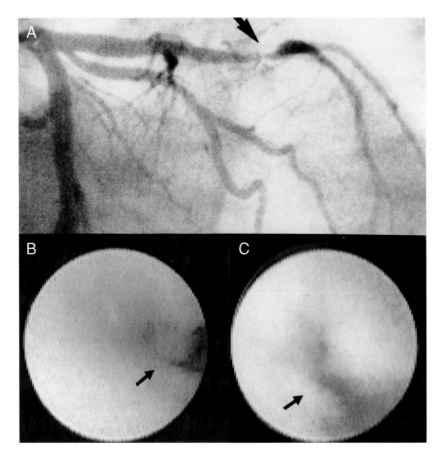

Fig. 18. K.K., 71-year-old male. Unstable angina pectoris. **A:** stenosis in the middle segment of the LAD (arrow). **B:** an obstructing flap in the same portion (arrow). **C:** red thrombus behind the flap (arrow).

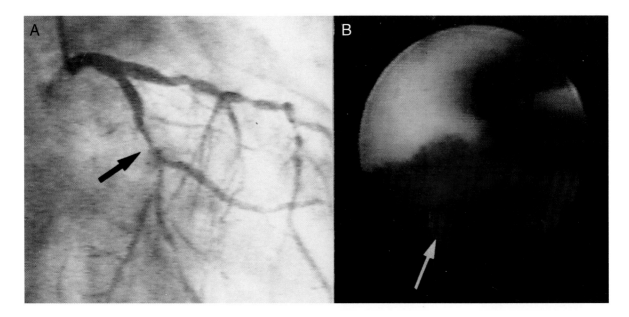

Fig. 19. C.E., 60-year-old female. Unstable angina pectoris. **A:** angiogram showing 99% stenosis in the middle segment of the LCx (arrow). **B:** streamer-like dark red thrombus in the segment just proximal to the most stenotic portion (arrow).

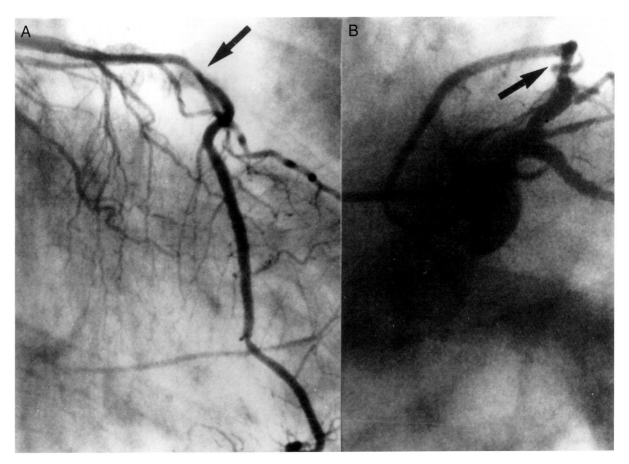

Fig. 20. R.K., 70-year-old male. Unstable angina pectoris. An insignificant stenosis in the middle segment of the LAD (arrows).

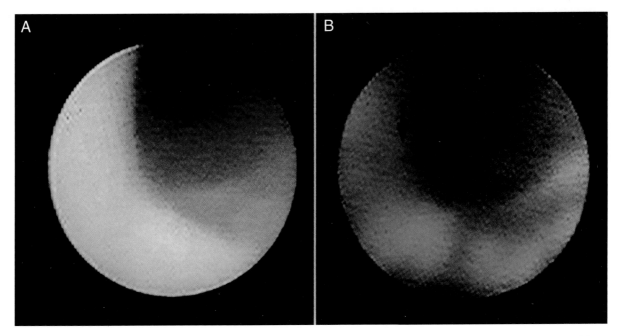

Fig. 21. The same patient as in Fig. 20. **A:** frosted glass-like luminal surface. **B:** diffuse staining with Evans blue.

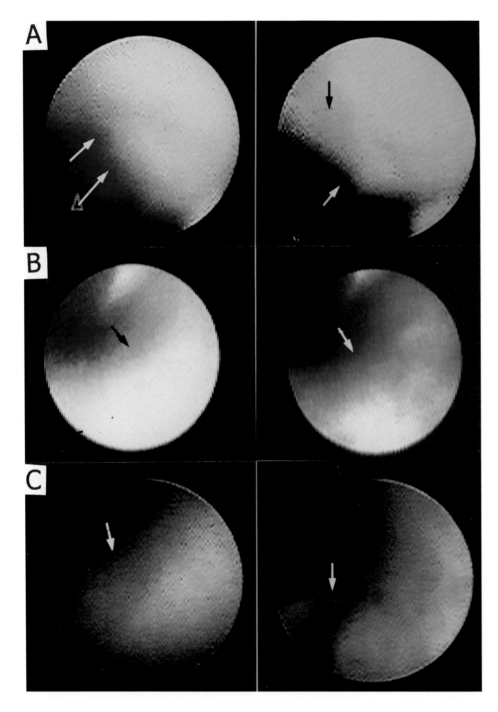

Fig. 22. Dye staining of the frosted glass-like coronary segments in unstable angina pectoris. **Left:** before Evans blue staining. **Right:** after staining. **A:** yellow plaque with focal staining (arrows). **B:** white plaque with diffuse Evans blue staining (white arrow). **C:** light yellow plaque with focal staining.

the same angioscopic appearance. It was revealed that multiple fibrin threads with platelet aggregates arising from the damaged endothelial cells, like sea grasses, induced this peculiar angioscopic appearance (see Chapter 9). Therefore, it is concluded that a frosted glass-like surface indicates that the remnant of thrombus remained after autolysis or detachment.

Ultrasonographically, there are no obvious differences in plaque characteristics except large disruption between unstable and stable angina pec-

toris.[17] Discrimination of a frosted glass-like surface is beyond conventional IVUS.

Acute Myocardial Infarction

Thrombus

Complex plaque with thrombus is found in the majority of patients with acute myocardial infarction.

Fig. 23 shows coronary angiographic, angioscopic, and IVUS images of the obstructed RCA obtained 2 hours after the onset of attack in a patient with acute myocardial infarction. A red thrombus mixed with yellow glistening matter occupied the proximal segment of the RCA. Echolucent cavities in the culprit soft plaque were detected by IVUS performed after thrombolysis.

Fig. 24 shows obstruction of the proximal segment of the RCA with white and globular thrombus.

Fig. 25 shows a long streamer-like thrombus

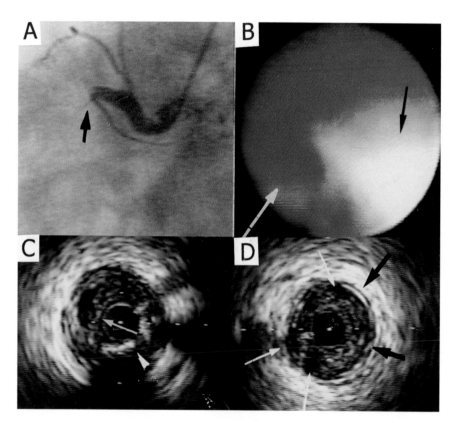

Fig. 23. Y.U., 68-year-old male. Acute myocardial infarction. **A:** obstruction in the proximal segment of the RCA (arrow). **B:** red thrombus (white arrow) and glistening yellow matter (black arrow) occupying the lumen. **C:** proximal portion of the plaque. Arrow: cavity. Arrowhead: calcification. **D:** plaque at the most stenotic portion. Black arrows: external elastic lamina. White arrows: cavities.

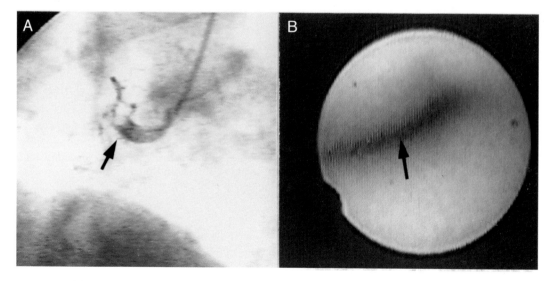

Fig. 24. E.I., 72-year-old male. Acute myocardial infarction. **A:** obstruction of the proximal segment of the RCA (arrow). **B:** smooth-surfaced white ball thrombus occupying the segment (arrow).

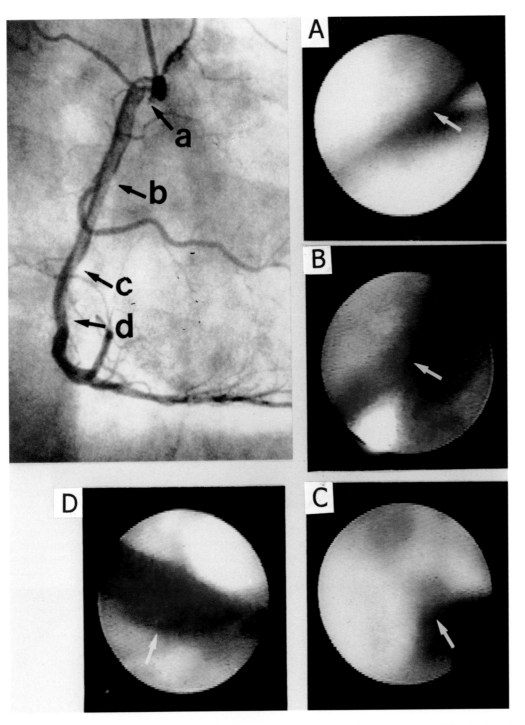

Fig. 25. J.F., 74-year-old male. Acute myocardial infarction. **A:** an angiogram showing a typical lead pipe sign, indicating existence of a streamer-like thrombus originating in the proximal segment and extending into the distal segment of the RCA. a–d in the angiogram, respectively, correspond to A–D in the angioscopic images.

identified by both angiography and angioscopy. Color of the thrombus differed from portion to portion.

Fig. 26 shows angiographic, IVUS, and angioscopic images of an ulcer. The ulcer was opacified with contrast material in the late phase of angiogra-

phy. The ulcer was partially covered with thin intima. This intima was thin and yellow by angioscopy. Exposed yellow atheromatous tissues with glittering small particles (calcium and/or cholesterol crystals) were observed in the bottom of the ulcer. The ulcer

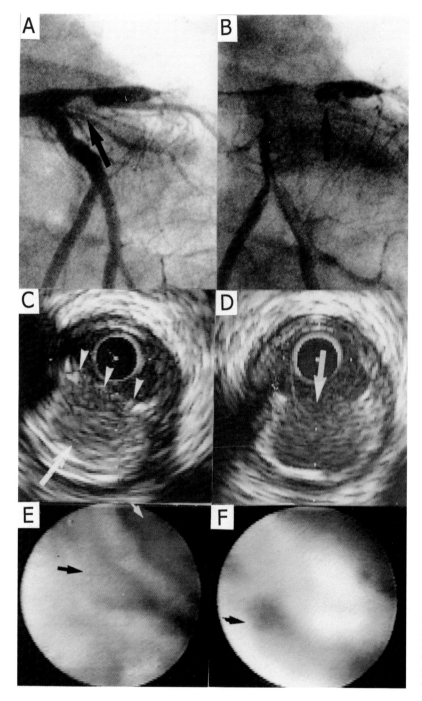

Fig. 26. K.I., 70-year-old male. Acute myocardial infarction. **A:** an eccentric plaque in the proximal segment of the LAD (arrow). **B:** an ulcer in the plaque (arrow). **C:** a large ulcer (arrow) covered with a thin intima (arrowheads). **D:** exposed ulcer (arrow). **E:** intima covering the ulcer (black arrow). White arrow: surrounding tissues (endothelial cells) stained with Evans blue. **F:** interior of the ulcer.

itself was not stained with Evans blue while the surrounding tissues were stained.

Configuration of Obstructed Coronary Stump and Color of Thrombus

Angiographically, the stumps of the obstructed coronary arteries in acute coronary syndromes are classified into hazy, concave (tapering), convex (protruding), and cut-off configurations. Cotton candy-

like white or pink thrombus was frequently observed in the hazy stump group and smooth-surfaced ball-like white thrombus was frequently observed in the convex stump group (Fig. 27; Table 1).

Presence or Absence of Thrombus and Color of Thrombus

The relationships between presence or absence of thrombus identified by angioscopy and angio-

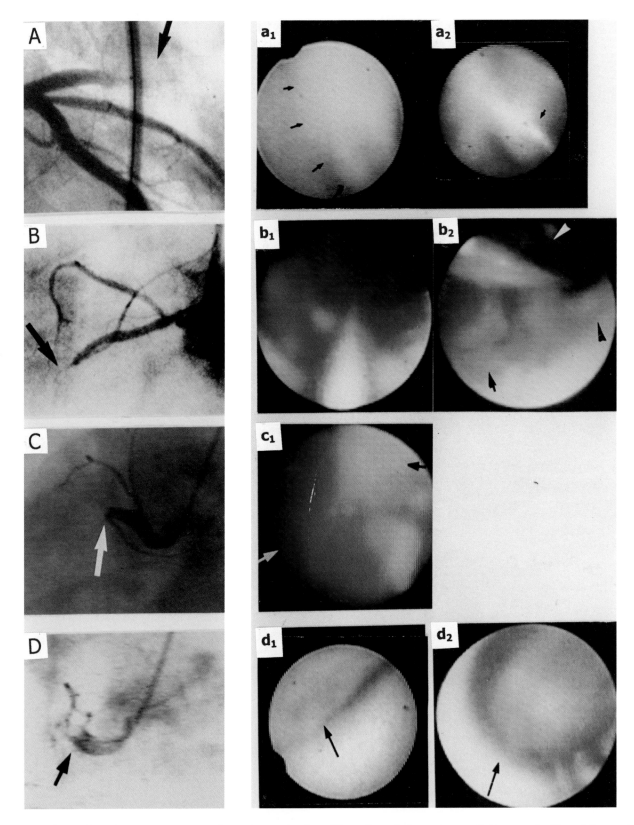

Fig. 27. Relationships between stump configuration and color of thrombus. **A:** hazy stump. Cotton candy-like white or pink thrombus by angioscopy. **B:** concave stump. Red obstructive thrombus or streamer-like thrombus arising from a prestenotic disrupted plaque and obstructing the most stenotic portion. **C:** cut-off stump. Red obstructive thrombus by angioscopy. **D:** convex stump. White or pink ball thrombus.

Table 1
Angiographic Coronary Stump Configuration and Thrombus

Angiographic Stump Configuration	No. of Stumps	Tight Globular Thrombus			Cotton Candy-like Thrombus		
		red	pink	white	red	pink	white
Cut-off	5	4	1				
Concave	6	5	1				
Convex	6		2	4			
Hazy	6				1	1	4

graphic changes were examined. It was revealed that TIMI grade had no relation to the presence or absence of thrombus. On the other hand, the time lag from the onset to angioscopy was shorter in the thrombus-present patients, suggesting that autolysis had occurred in the thrombus-absent group (Table 2).

Relationships between color of thrombus and angiographic changes were also examined. However, there were no relationships between TIMI grade and color of thrombus. On the other hand, time lag from the onset of attack to angioscopy was longer in the white thrombus group, indicating that dispersion of blood cells by autolysis or washout by the bloodstream contributed to thrombus color (Table 3) (see Chapter 9).

Table 2
Relationships Between Presence or Absence of Thrombus Examined by Angioscopy and Angiographic Changes

	Thrombus Present	Thrombus Absent
No. of Patients	27	14
Time after the onset of attack	4.1 ± 3.2*	5.6 ± 3.9
TIMI grade		
0	16	8
I	3	3
II	6	1
III	2	2
Angiographic filling defect	6*	0
Haziness	10*	0
Distance from proximal side branch	5.1 ± 3.4*	3.6 ± 3.8

P < 0.05 vs. thrombus absent.

Glistening Yellow Matter in the Disrupted Plaque and Glistening Yellow Rim of the Disrupted Plaque

Glistening yellow matter was often observed in the disrupted plaque. Our ex-vivo microscopic study revealed that calcium and cholesterol crystals in the atheromatous tissues are responsible for glistening (see Chapter 5). Also, the proximal nondisrupted rim glistened, indicating that these substances are seen through the endothelium (Figs. 28, 29).

Dye Image Angioscopy in Acute Myocardial Infarction

Based on ex-vivo study (see Chapter 9), dye image angioscopy with Evans blue was performed to

Table 3
Relationship Between Thrombus Color and Time Lag After the Onset of Attack

	Thrombus Color			
	red	white	pink or mixed	thrombus absent
No. of patients	8	8	11	14
Time after onset of attack(s)	3.9 ± 2.1	4.9 ± 5.5*	3.7 ± 2.0	5.6 ± 3.9
TIMI grade (>II)	1	1	3	4

*P<0.05 vs. red.

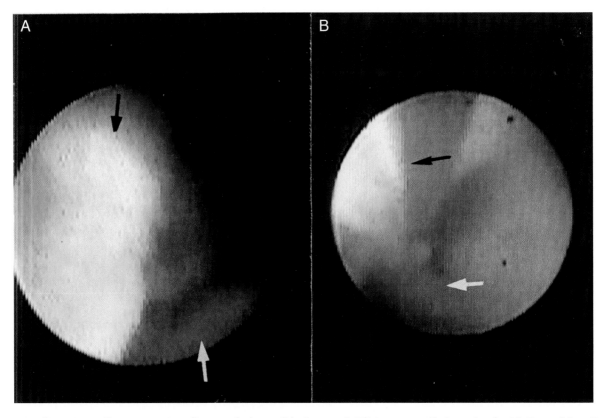

Fig. 28. A: Glistening yellow matter in a disrupted plaque (black arrow). White arrow: fibrin stained with Evans blue. **B:** glistening yellow rim of a disrupted plaque (black arrow). White arrow: red thrombus on the disrupted portion.

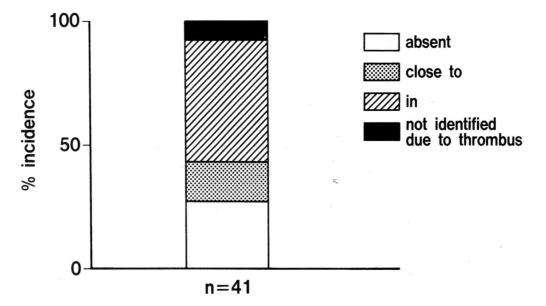

Fig. 29. Incidence of glistening yellow matter in the disrupted plaques and that of glistening yellow rims of disrupted plaques in patients with acute myocardial infarction.

Table 4
Dye Image Angioscopy of Disrupted Plaques With Evans Blue in Acute Myocardial Infarction

	No.	Stained	Not Stained
Flap	13	11	2
Ulcer	8		8
Lipid core	7		7
Fibrous cap	8	7	1
Thrombus			
red	11		11
mixed	5	1	4
white	3	3	

discriminate substances composing the disrupted plaques.

The majority of flaps and fibrous caps covering the culprit plaques were stained, indicating that the endothelial cells attached to the flaps and those covering the culprit plaques were damaged. The exposed atheromatous tissues and the interior of the ulcer that is composed of exposed atheromatous tissues were not stained, indicating that atheromatous tissues have no affinity to this dye. White thrombus was stained but red ones were not stained, indicating that the former is composed mainly of fibrin (Table 4).

Old Myocardial Infarction and Post-Infarction Angina

In patients with old myocardial infarction, complex plaques with thrombus are frequently observed (Fig. 4).

One to 3 months after the onset of acute myocardial infarction in patients who had not undergone coronary interventions, the plaques that were considered culprit for the attacks were observed by angioscopy. Fig. 30 shows an eccentric and overhanging plaque detected by angiography in the middle segment of the RCA in a patient with post-infarction angina. Angioscopically, the plaque was brownish yellow, irregular, and protruded into the lumen and had a small red thrombus on it. Probably, the atheromatous tissues were not lost during disruption and blood turbulence caused by it resulted in recurrent thrombus formation, leading to anginal attacks.

In the chronic stage, the plaques that were responsible for acute myocardial infarction are classified into those in which atheromatous tissues are not lost, those partially lost, and those almost completely lost showing dormant volcano-like configuration (Fig. 31). According to our study in a small number of patients, there was a tendency that post-infarction angina was more frequently associated with the plaques in which exposed atheromatous tissues were

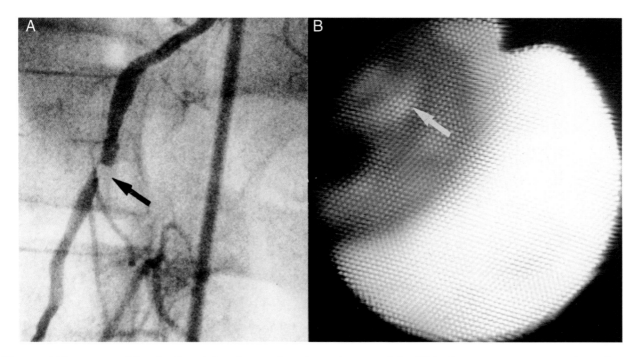

Fig. 30. A.T., 70-year-old male. Post-infarction angina. **A:** angiogram of the RCA. Arrow: an eccentric and overhanging plaque. **B:** angioscopic appearance of the same plaque. Arrow: thrombus.

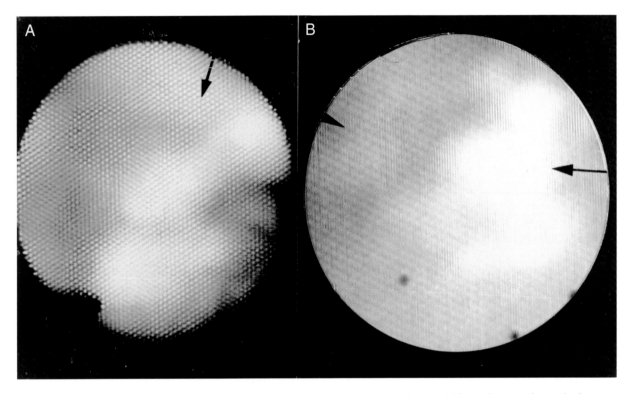

Fig. 31. A: disrupted plaque in which atheromatous tissues are almost retained. **B:** a delle, indicating loss of atheromatous tissues (arrowhead) surrounded by a glistening yellow rim (inactive volcano-like) (arrow).

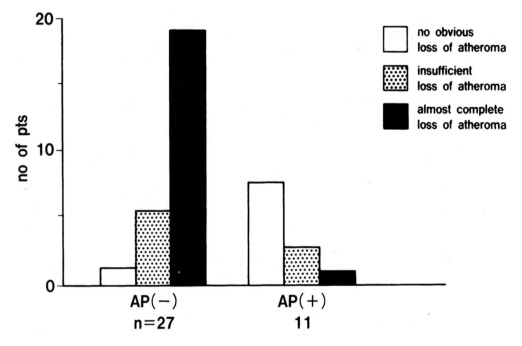

Fig. 32. Relationship between post-infarction angina and plaque configuration.

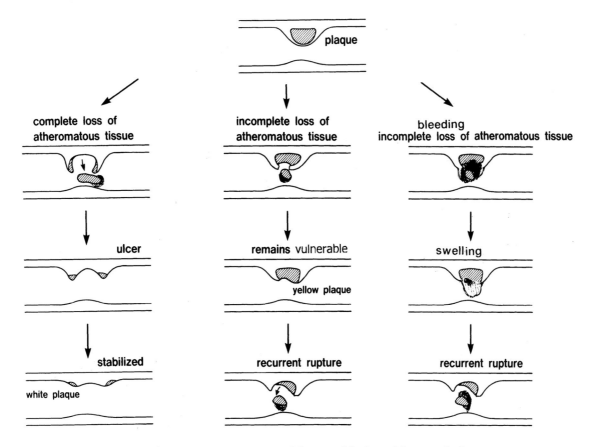

Fig. 33. Schematic representation of the possible fate of disrupted plaques.

not lost, suggesting the different fate of the disrupted plaques (Figs. 32, 33).

Lurking Thrombus in the Segment Proximal to the Angiographic Culprit Plaque for Acute Coronary Syndromes

In 10% to 30% of patients with acute coronary syndromes, the plaques angiographically culprit (the plaque occupying the most stenotic portion) for the attacks are angioscopically apparently intact (Fig. 1).

In addition to endothelial damage detectable only by dye image angioscopy, we occasionally found a thrombus not at the angiographically culprit plaque but in a nonstenotic segment proximal to and clearly separated from the angiographically culprit plaque.

Fig. 34 shows obstruction of the middle segment of the LAD in a patient with acute myocardial infarc-

tion. Angioscopically, the plaque located at the obstructed portion was light yellow and almost intact. However, a glistening yellow and irregular plaque was found in a segment angiographically not stenotic and several millimeters proximal to the former plaque. In addition, a streamer-like red thrombus mixed with brown matter originated from the plaque and extended into the angiographic culprit plaque. The plaque and thrombus were not detectable by angiography.

Fig. 35 also shows obstruction of the proximal segment of the LAD in a patient with unstable angina pectoris. Careful observation of angiograms revealed a small ball-like negative shadow in a segment approximately 3 mm proximal to the obstructed portion. Angioscopy revealed that the shadow was due to a ball-like brown mass that originated in a nonstenotic portion and extended into the angiographically obstructed portion. However, it was not determined whether the brown mass was an organized thrombus or atheromatous debris ejected from the disrupted proximal plaque.

Fig. 36 shows obstruction in the proximal seg-

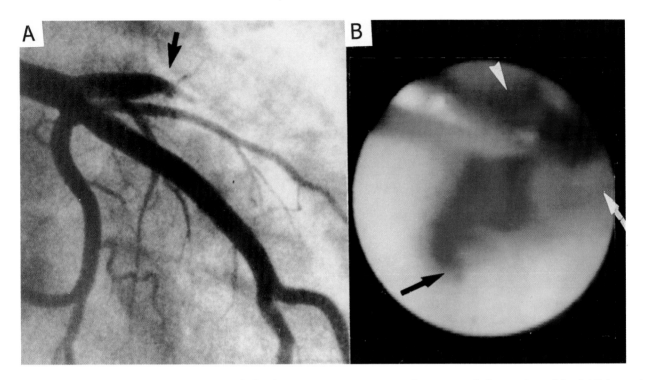

Fig. 34. A.K., 76-year-old male. Acute myocardial infarction. **A:** an angiogram showing total obstruction of the LAD (arrow). **B:** angioscopic image of the obstructed portion in the LAD. Black arrow: a streamer-like red thrombus mixed with brown matter arising from a glistening yellow disrupted plaque in a nonstenotic portion and extending distally (arrowhead) to obstruct the angiographically most stenotic distal portion (white arrow).

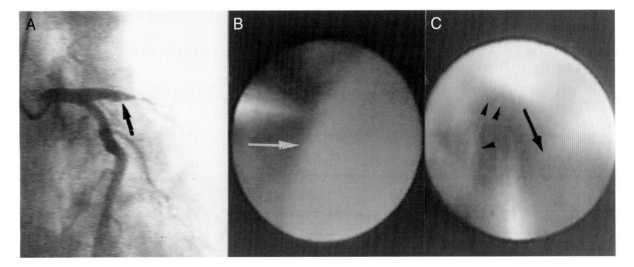

Fig. 35. K.Y., 69-year-old male. Unstable angina pectoris. **A:** angiographic image. A small ball-like negative shadow in the LAD just proximal to the obstructed portion (arrow). **B:** angioscopic image. A ball-like brown mass corresponding to the shadow in A. **C:** observation of the same brown mass from more proximal portion. Arrow: the mass that extended into the angiographically obstructed portion (arrowheads).

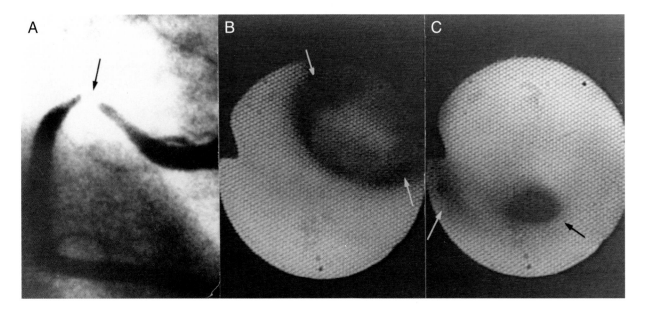

Fig. 36. M.T., 77-year-old female. Stable angina pectoris. **A:** obstruction at the proximal segment of the RCA (arrow). **B:** a doughnut-like dark red thrombus (white arrows) just proximal to a white regular plaque (**C**).

ment of the RCA. Angioscopy revealed a doughnut-like thrombus just proximal to a white, regular, concentric plaque. Thus, we frequently found a prestenotic thrombus that was angiographically not detectable (Table 5). Therefore, we call this thrombus a "lurking thrombus."

In order to gain insight into the underlying mechanism(s) for the lurking thrombus, we performed perfusion of removed atherosclerotic human coronary artery with canine arterial blood. It was revealed that a doughnut-like thrombus is rapidly formed proximal to the plaque.[18] It is well known that such a thrombus is formed due to prestenotic blood turbulence. We also performed a chronic experiment in which a canine coronary artery was

stenosed by transcatheter implantation of a water-absorbable resin. Angioscopy performed 2 weeks later revealed red, yellow, or brown masses just proximal to the stenotic portion. Histological studies revealed red, yellow, and brown masses were, respectively, fresh, organizing, and organized thrombi.

Based on this and previous experiments, we recognize that at least 3 mechanisms may participate in the prestenotic lurking thrombus: antegrade growth of thrombus from the disrupted plaque at the stenotic portion (Fig. 37A), thrombus growth from the disrupted nonstenotic plaque that is located proximal to the stenotic portion (Fig. 37B), and prestenotic thrombus growth due to rheological mechanisms (Fig. 37C).

Table 5
Prestenotic Lurking Thrombus

| Coronary Syndromes | No. of Patients | Lurking Thrombus | | | | Originated from Prestenotic Plaque | Detectable by Angiography |
		red	brown	mixed	total (%)		
SAP	50	2 (1)*	1		3 (6.0)	1	
UAP	42	3	2	3	8 (19.0)	2	1
AMI	44	2	4	3	9 (20.4)	3	2
OMI	20	1	3	1	5 (25.0)	1	2

*Dark red in 1 patient, SAP: stable angina pectoris. UAP: unstable angina pectoris. AMI: acute myocardial infarction. OMI: old myocardial infarction (over 1 month after the attack).

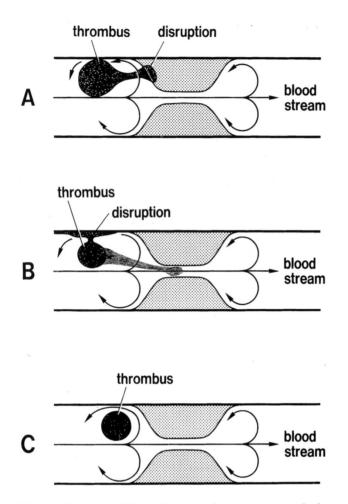

Fig. 37. Three possible mechanisms for a prestenotic lurking thrombus. **A:** antegrade thrombus growth from the disrupted plaque. **B:** disruption of a plaque located in an angiographically nonstenotic proximal portion and thrombus growth from it extending distally into the angiographically obstructed portion. **C:** formation of a doughnut-like thrombus just proximal to the plaque due to blood turbulence.

Angiographic Tandem Coronary Lesion and Its Rheological Mechanism

Angiographically, more than 2 stenoses in a series are not infrequently observed in the same coronary segment. These lesions are called "tandem lesions" since they resemble tandem. It is generally thought that the individual lesions that constitute tandem lesions are independently developed atherosclerotic plaques.

Angioscopically, individual narrowing of angiographically documented tandem lesions appeared only as a tangentally expressed prominent portion of

an atherosclerotic spiral fold (Fig. 38). The directions of the fold were counterclockwise in the proximal to middle segments and clockwise in the distal segment of the RCA, clockwise in the proximal to middle segments and counterclockwise in the distal segment of the LAD, and counterclockwise in the proximal to middle segments of the LCx (Table 6). The bloodstream always ran along the spiral folds in the tandem lesions (Fig. 39).[19]

Shear stress on the vascular wall enhances the release of vasoactive substances from the endothelium[20] and enhances uptake by the endothelium such as low density lipoprotein.[21] Deposition of lipids occurs in the region of flow separation and in regions with low shear stress, resulting in atherosclerotic stenosis.[22] Therefore, it is likely that spiral laminal flow induces spiral folds. It is likely that such shallow spiral folds grow into angiographically demonstrable tandem lesions. We found by intracardiac ultrasound system (ICUS) that spiral laminal flow is generated by the left ventricle (Fig. 40). Flow patterns of the bloodstream from the aorta into the coronary artery may be different among the 3 major coronary arteries, leading to different directions of spiral folds. A possible process of formation of a tandem coronary lesion is shown in Fig. 41. The direction of the spiral fold in the distal segment is opposite to that seen in the proximal to middle segments. In the coronary artery, the major inflow occurs during diastole, while backflow occurs during systole. This backflow may have modified the direction of the spiral fold in the distal segment. Since individual stenosis of a tandem lesion is the most prominent portion of a spiral atherosclerotic plaque, dissection of one prominent portion may result in a long spiral dissection that is experienced during intervention. Therefore, in case of intervention in the tandem lesion, this anatomic evidence should be taken into consideration.

Coronary Spasm

Coronary vasospasm is induced spontaneously or provoked by exercise and drugs such as ergonovine maleate and acetylcholine. It is generally believed that the less atherosclerotic portion of eccentric stenosis contracts, resulting in a slit-like obstruction.[23–25]

Fig. 42 shows spasm in the distal segment of the LAD induced by intracoronary injection of ergonovine maleate. Before spasm provocation, the segment was white and smooth and the lumen was almost round.

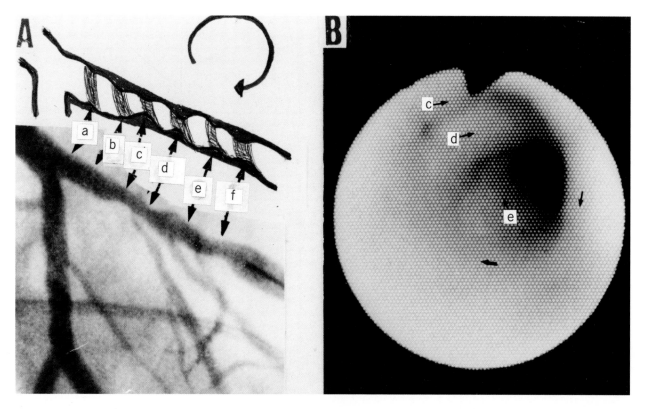

Fig. 38. Tandem lesion in the LAD. **A:** angiographic image and its schematic representation. **B:** angioscopic image of the same tandem lesion. c, d, e in B correspond to those in A, respectively.

On provocation of spasm, the lumen became slit-like, compressing the 0. 014-inch guidewire. We observed slit-like obstructions in 5 of 6 patients and concentric obstruction in the remaining 1 patient.

Coronary Squeezing (Myocardial Bridging)

The major coronary arteries pass over the epicardial surface. In 5–12% of humans, short coronary segments descend into the myocardium for a variable distance.[26] Because a bridge of myocardium passes over the involved coronary segment, systolic contraction can cause narrowing of the segment, namely "coronary squeezing." When squeezing is severe, blood flow may be decreased, resulting in myocardial ischemia and atypical symptoms. This phenomenon is enhanced by nitroglycerin through augmentation of myocardial contraction due to reflex sympathetic excitation.

Fig. 43 shows systolic luminal narrowing of the distal segment of the LAD due to squeezing. It is noted that the endothelium at the inlet of the squeezed segment is damaged due to blood turbulence, and thrombus is formed on it, resulting in acute coronary syndromes (Fig. 44).

Table 6
Direction of Spiral Folds in Angiographically Documented Tandem Lesions

	RCA		LAD		LCX	
	proximal to	mid-distal	proximal to	mid-distal	proximal to	mid-distal
Clockwise	0/9	1/6	9/12	1/7	1/8	1/2
Counter clockwise	9/9	5/6	2/12*	6/7	7/8	1/2

*Unclear in 1.

RCA: right coronary artery. LAD: left anterior descending. LCX: left circumflex.

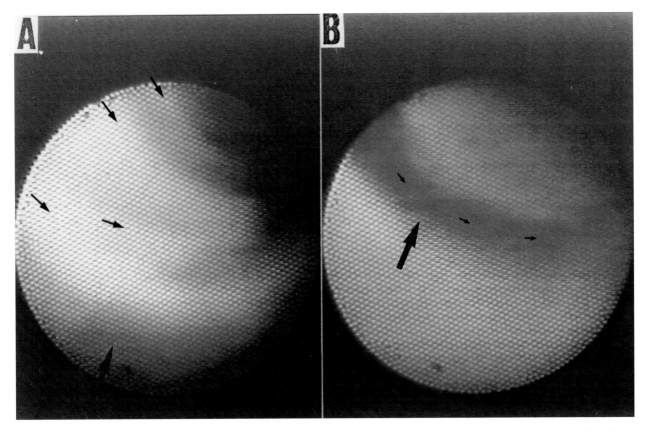

Fig. 39. A: spiral folds (small arrows) and bloodstream (large arrow) in the proximal segment of the RCA. **B:** bloodstream moved to the next fold (large arrow).

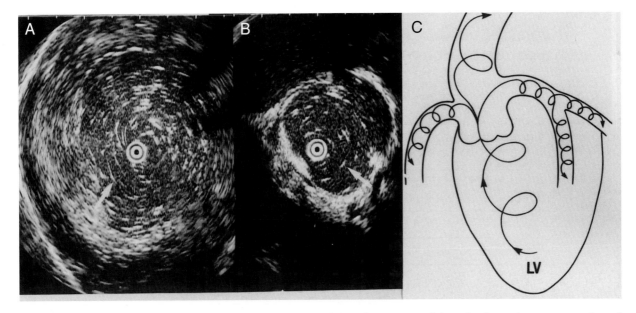

Fig. 40. ICUS images of bloodstream in the canine left ventricle (**A**) and aortic root (**B**), and schematic representation of spiral bloodstream (**C**). Arrows: bloodstream visualized with air microbubbles.

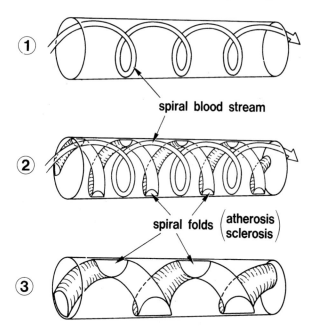

spiral blood stream

spiral folds (atherosis / sclerosis)

CAG

stenoses

Fig. 41. Schematic representation of possible process of formation of tandem coronary lesion.

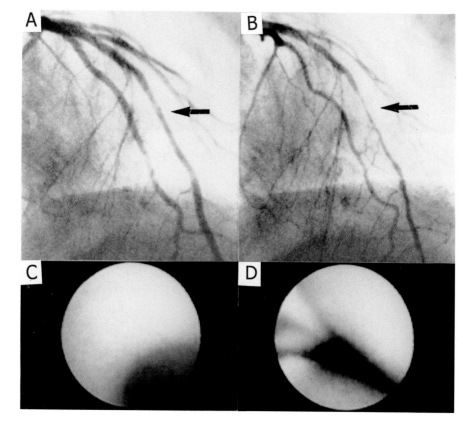

Fig. 42. S.K., 63-year-old male. Vasospastic angina pectoris. **A** and **B**: angiograms before and during vasospasm induced by intracoronary injection of ergonovine maleate, respectively. Arrow: spasm. **C** and **D**: angioscopic images of the coronary segment corresponding to that indicated by an arrow in B before and during vasospasm, respectively.

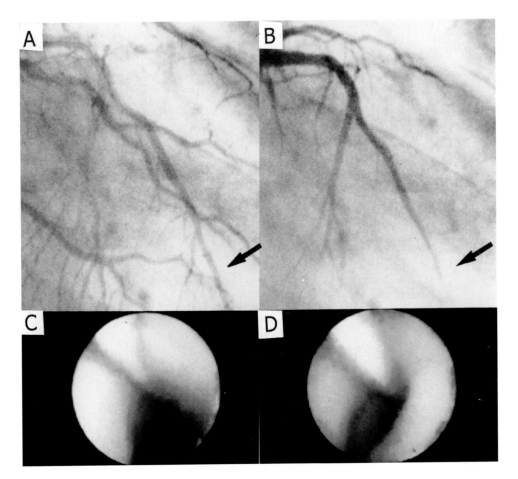

Fig. 43. K.K., 60-year-old male. Coronary squeezing. **A** and **B**: coronary angiograms during diastole and systole, respectively. Arrow: squeezing. **C** and **D**: angioscopic images during diastole and systole, respectively.

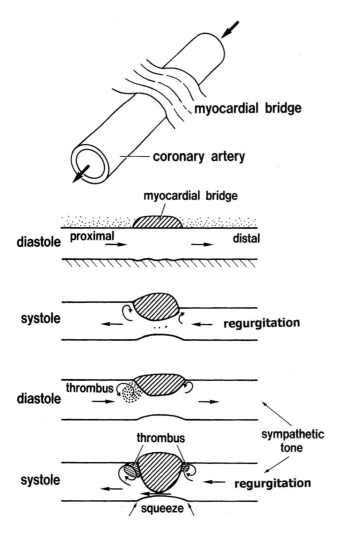

Fig. 44. Possible mechanisms for thrombus formation induced by squeezing.

References

1. Fuster V, Badimon L, Badimon JJ, et al: The pathogenesis of coronary artery disease and acute coronary syndromes. N Engl J Med 326:242–250, 1992.
2. Thieme T, Wernecke KD, Meyer R, et al: Angioscopic evaluation of atherosclerotic plaques: Validation by histomorphology analysis and associations with stable and unstable coronary syndromes. J Am Coll Cardiol 28:1–6, 1996.
3. Silva JA, Escobar AE, Collins TJ, et al: Unstable angina: A comparison of angioscopic findings between diabetic and nondiabetic patients. Circulation 42:1731–1736, 1995.
4. Frink RJ: Chronic ulcerated plaques: New insight into the pathogenesis of acute coronary disease. J Invas Cardiol 6:173–185, 1994.
5. de Fyter PJ, Ozaki Y, Baptista J, et al: Ischemia-related lesion characteristics in patients with stable or unstable angina. Circulation 92:1408–1413, 1995.
6. Waxman S, Mittleman MA, Zarich SW, et al: Angioscopic assessment of coronary lesions underlying thrombus. Am J Cardiol 79:1106–1109, 1997.
7. Uchida Y: Percutaneous coronary angioscopy. Jpn Heart J 33:271–294, 1992.
8. Uchida Y: Angioscopic detection of vulnerable coronary plaques and prediction of acute coronary syndromes. In: The Vulnerable Atherosclerotic Plaques. Fuster V (ed). Futura Publishing Co, Armonk, NY, 1999, pp 111–129.
9. Mizuno K, Miyamoto A, Satomura K: Angioscopic coronary macromorphology in patients with acute coronary syndromes. Lancet 337:809–812, 1991.
10. Yamada K, Fujimori Y, Morio H, et al: Characteristics of the culprit coronary lesions and estimation of the interventional treatments in patients. J Am Coll Cardiol 33(Suppl A):64A, 1999 (abstract).
11. Morio H, Fujimori Y, Terasawa K, et al: Evaluation of culprit coronary plaques by dye image angioscopy. Jpn Circ J 64(Suppl I):203, 2000.

12. Uchida Y, Nakamura F, Tomaru T, et al: Prediction of acute coronary syndromes by percutaneous coronary angioscopy in patients with stable angina. Am Heart J 130:195–203, 1995.

13. Falk E: Unstable angina with fatal outcome: Dynamic coronary thrombosis leading to infarction and/or sudden death. Circulation 71:699–708, 1985.

14. Uchida Y, Murao S: Cyclic fluctuations in coronary blood pressure and flow induced by coronary artery occlusion. Jpn Heart J 16:454–464, 1975.

15. Uchida Y, Uchida Y, Murao S: Angiographic changes associated with recurring reduction of carotid and cerebral blood flow. Jpn Circ J 45:424–437, 1981.

16. Farb A, Burke AP, Tang AL, et al: Coronary plaque erosion without rupture into a lipid core. Circulation 93:1354–1363, 1996.

17. Honne J, Saito A, Kammatsuse K: Culprit plaques in unstable angina. Coronary 15:84–89, 1998 (in Japanese).

18. Uchida Y, Tomaru T, Sumino S, et al: Fiberoptic observation of thrombosis and thrombolysis in isolated human coronary artery. Am Heart J 112:694–696, 1986.

19. Uchida Y, Nakamura F, Tomaru T, et al: Rheological significance of tandem lesions of the coronary artery. Heart Vessels 10:106–110, 1995.

20. Frangos JA: Flow effects on prostacyclin production by cultured human endothelial cells. Science 227:1477–1479, 1985.

21. Spraque EA: Influence of steady-state fluid-imposed wall shear stress on the binding, internalization and degradation of low density lipoproteins by cultured arterial endothelium. Circulation 76:648–656, 1987.

22. Caro CG, Fitz-Gerald JM, Schroter RC: Atheroma and arterial wall shear: Observation, correlation and proposal for a shear-dependent mass transfer mechanism for atherogenesis. Proc R Soc Lond 117:109–159, 1971.

23. Isner JM, Fortin AH, Fortin RV: Depletion of smooth muscle from the media of atherosclerotic coronary arteries: A potential factor in the pathogenesis of myocardial ischemia and the variable response to antianginal therapy. Clin Res 31:193A, 1983 (abstract).

24. Factor SM, Cho S: Smooth muscle contraction band in the media of coronary arteries: A postmortem marker of antemortem coronary spasm? J Am Coll Cardiol 6:1329–1337, 1983.

25. Saner HE, Gobel FL, Salmonowitz E, et al: The disease-free wall in coronary atherosclerosis: Its relation to degree of obstruction. J Am Coll Cardiol 6:1096–1099, 1985.

26. Kramer JR, Kitazume H, Proudtit WL, Sones FM Jr: Clinical significance of isolated coronary bridges: Benign and frequent condition involving the left anterior descending artery. Am Heart J 103:282–286, 1982.

Chapter 13

Specific Coronary Diseases

Kawasaki Disease

Kawasaki disease (mucocutaneous lymphnode syndrome) was first described by Kawasaki in Japan in 1967. It is a generalized vasculitis of unknown etiology.[1,2] Eighty percent of cases occur in children under 5 years of age. Coronary artery abnormalities develop in approximately 20% of untreated patients. In these children, aneurysms of the coronary arteries with narrowing, tortuosity, and obstruction develop. In cases with giant aneurysms, intracoronary thrombosis, stenosis, and myocardial infarction can occur.[3-5] Myocardial infarction occurs 2–6 weeks after the onset of symptoms. Postmortem examination revealed a 25–35% incidence of myocardial infarction.[1] Processes of aneurysm formation, thrombosis, fibrotic thickening and resultant obstruction, and recanalization are shown in Fig. 1.

We followed up 6 patients who had giant coronary aneurysms by angiography for 8–13 years, and when they were 9 years or older, percutaneous coronary angioscopy and IVUS were performed.[6]

Fig. 2 shows giant aneurysms in both the right coronary artery (RCA) and the left anterior descending (LAD) artery, which were observed in a 12-year-old boy with acute myocardial infarction that occurred 8 years after the onset of disease. Angioscopy revealed a red thrombus in the RCA that corresponded to the defect (Fig. 3A). Six months later, the thrombus still remained although its color changed into reddish brown (Fig. 3B). One year after the initial angioscopy, the thrombus became yellow, indicating organization (Fig. 3C). Angiography performed 2 years later revealed that the aneurysm in the RCA was calcified and diffuse narrowing developed with massive antegrade collaterals (Fig. 4B). IVUS revealed thick fibrous tissues surrounding the narrowed lumen where the aneurysm existed (Fig. 5A). Angioscopy revealed a white luminal surface with a patch of yellow (Fig. 5B) and new formation of small vessels (Fig. 5C).

During angiographic and angioscopic follow-up for 8–13 years in 6 patients, aneurysm disappeared in 5, narrowing developed in all, and acute myocardial infarction developed in 4 patients. Among them, 2 patients underwent coronary artery bypass grafting (CABG) with saphenous vein grafts. The grafted native arteries were obstructed in all of them. Fortunately, however, the obstructed native artery was recanalized by neovascularization in one. Fig. 6 shows obstruction of a native artery after CABG. The obstructed portion was white and the remnants of obstructed branches were observed. Except for a localized yellow patch in 1 patient, the luminal surface of the aneurysms and stenotic coronary segments remained white during angioscopic follow-up.

Aortitis Syndrome

Aortitis syndrome is a unique inflammatory cardiovascular disease of unknown origin and is observed in Asian women. This disease affects the aorta and its large branches. The adventitia and media are affected and secondary changes in the intima develop, resulting in stenoses or dilatation and calcification of the adventitia. Involvement of the coronary artery is rarely observed.

Fig. 7 shows angiographic, angioscopic, and IVUS images of the stenotic middle segment of the LCx in a patient with this syndrome. Angioscopically, the luminal surface was smooth and white. IVUS revealed concentric stenosis with calcification of the media and adventitia. We observed stenotic coronary segments in 3 patients with this disease. All of the segments were white and smooth. However, angioscopic differentiation from other categories of disease was difficult. Identification of adventitial calcification is one important finding for diagnosis of this disease.

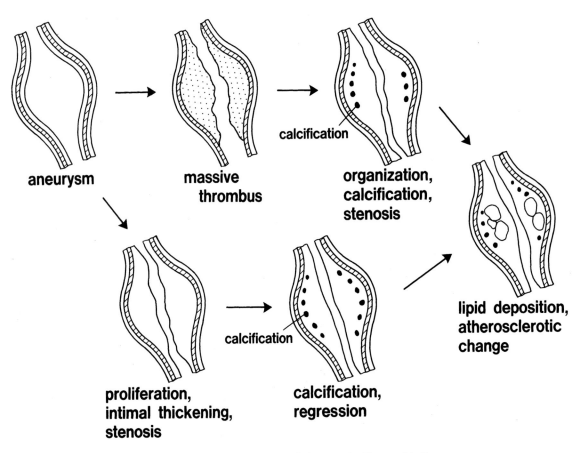

Fig. 1. Process of coronary arterial changes in Kawasaki disease.

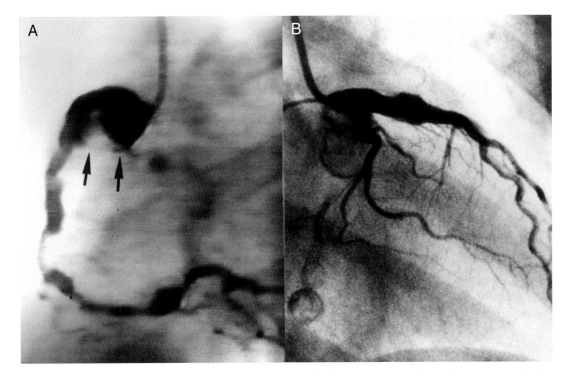

Fig. 2. A.K., 13-year-old male. Kawasaki disease. Giant aneurysms in both the RCA and the LAD. Arrows: a defect suggesting thrombus.

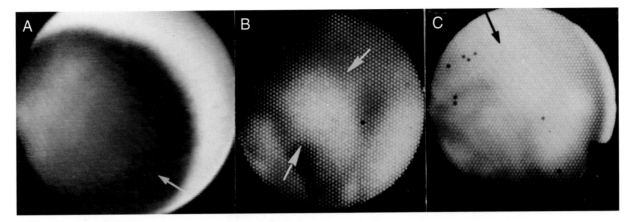

Fig. 3. The same patient as in Fig. 1. **A:** red and globular thrombus that corresponded to the defect in Fig. 1. **B:** the same thrombus 6 months later. **C:** the same thrombus 1 year later.

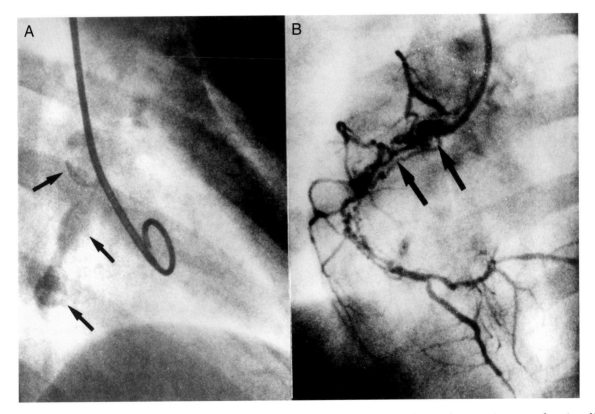

Fig. 4. The same patient as in Fig. 1. Two years later. **A:** calcification of aneurysm (arrows). **B:** angiograms showing diffuse narrowing and antegrade collaterals (arrows).

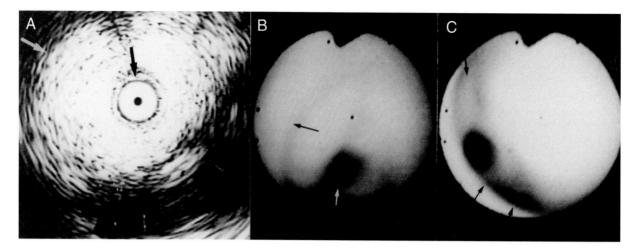

Fig. 5. The proximal segment of the RCA where the aneurysm had existed. **A:** IVUS image. Black arrow: residual lumen. White arrow: thick fibrotic tissues. **B:** yellow patch (black arrow) and residual lumen (white arrow). **C:** a few millimeters distal to B. Recanalized lumen due to neovascularization (arrows).

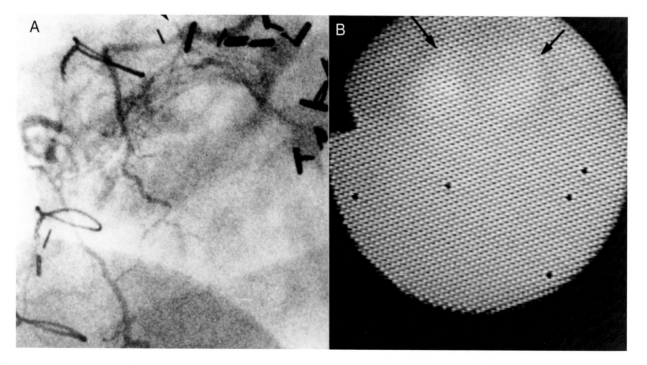

Fig. 6. Y.H., 15-year-old female. Old myocardial infarction. One year after CABG to the LAD and the RCA. **A:** angiogram showing obstruction of the RCA (arrow). **B:** angioscopic image of the obstructed portion. Arrows: remnant of obstructed lumen.

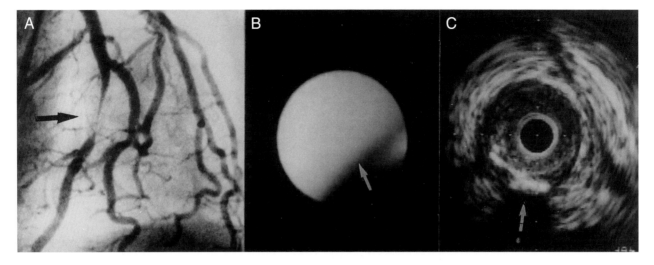

Fig. 7. Y.H., 45-year-old female. Aortitis syndrome. Angiographic (**A**), angioscopic (**B**), and IVUS (**C**) images of the middle segment of the LAD. Arrow in A: white plaque. Arrow in C: calcification in the adventitia and media.

References

1. Kawasaki T: Kawasaki Disease. Nankodo Co., Tokyo, 1988, pp 68–70.
2. Dajani AS, Taubert KA, Gerber MA: Diagnosis and therapy of Kawasaki disease in children. Circulation 87:1776, 1993.
3. Kato H, Ichinose E, Kawasaki T: Myocardial infarction in Kawasaki disease: Clinical analysis in 195 cases. J Pediatr 108:923–928, 1986.
4. Hiraishi S, Yashio K, Oguchi K, et al: Clinical course of cardiovascular involvement in the mucocutaneous lymphnode syndrome. Am J Cardiol 47:323, 1981.
5. Kato H, Ichinose E, Matsunaga S: Fate of coronary aneurysms in Kawasaki disease: Serial coronary angiography and long-term follow-up study. Am J Cardiol 49:1758–1761, 1982.
6. Ishikawa H, Sasaki M, Uchida Y, et al: Angioscopic observation of coronary lesions in Kawasaki disease. Circulation 84(Suppl):II-54, 1991.

Chapter 14

Coronary Luminal Changes Associated With Coronary Interventions

Angioscopic changes associated with intracoronary interventions were described for the first time by Uchida et al.[1] The acute and chronic changes following interventions are different among the plaques and therefore between stable angina and acute coronary syndromes, and also among the modalities of interventions. Complications are also different among different coronary syndromes and modalities of interventions.

Plain Old Balloon Coronary Angioplasty (POBA)

The changes in the coronary atherosclerotic plaques induced by POBA are largely influenced by the plaque structure, balloon size, and balloon pressure. Angioscopically, POBA-induced plaque changes are classified into minor and major changes. Minor changes are uneven surface and endothelial exfoliation. Histologically, the former is due to endothelial damages and erosion. However, these changes are hardly detectable by angiography and IVUS. The major changes are dissections, which are variously described as split, cleft, crack, fissure, fracture, intimal flap, bleeding, and thrombus. Bleeding is either purplish red or fresh red in color.[2] The former indicates venous bleeding and the latter, arterial bleeding. In addition to these changes, ejection of lipid pool debris, including lipids, calcium, and cholesterol crystals into the lumen should be added, since they are sometimes very dirty in color and mixed with thrombus and may cause distal embolism. Histologically, the depth of dissection is classified into 3 types (Table 1).[3] However, estimation of the depth of dissection is beyond angioscopy. IVUS is feasible for assessments of POBA-induced changes in deeper layers.

By IVUS, POBA-induced changes are classified into minor changes such as uneven surface and derangement of plaque frame, and major changes such as dissection confined to the intima, dissection extending to the media, and thrombus formation (Table 2). IVUS is not feasible for identification of thrombus.

Acute Changes

Stable Angina Pectoris

Fig. 1 shows angiographic changes in the stenotic middle segment of the left anterior descending (LAD) artery induced by POBA in a patient with stable angina. Angiographically, POBA resulted in sufficient and smooth luminal dilatation. Before POBA, the plaque at its most stenotic portion was light yellow in color and eccentric in configuration. However, the proximal rim was yellow with a mural red thrombus. By IVUS, the plaque at its most stenotic portion was eccentric and iso- to low echoic, namely, mixed. First dilatation caused a deep cleft and exposure of glistening yellow matter. Repeated dilatation resulted in sufficient dilatation with round configuration by both angioscopy and IVUS (Fig. 2).

Fig. 3 shows representative examples of POBA-induced changes in the plaques: a tear of membranous plaque, splitting of a globular plaque, and recanalization of an occlusive plaque.

Fig. 4 shows representative IVUS changes of the plaques induced by POBA: dissection confined to the intima, that extending to media, multiple dissection and separation of the intima from media.

Table 1
**Angioscopic Classification of POBA-Induced Changes in the
Culprit Plaques and Their Correlations to Histological Changes**

Angioscopic Changes	*Histological Changes*

A. Minor changes
   Uneven surface
   Endothelial exfoliation
   Erosion	

B. Major changes
  1) Dissection
    Split
    Cleft
    Crack
    Fissure
    Intimal flap
    Fracture
    Ejected lipid pool contents
  2) Bleeding and thrombosis
    Venous bleeding
    Arterial bleeding
    Red thrombus
    White thrombus
    Mixed thrombus
    Mixture of thrombus and atheromatous tissues
	Type I. Functional changes in the endothelial cells
	    without morphologic changes
	Type II. Endothelial denudation and intimal damages
	    but internal elastic lamina and media are intact
	
	Type III. Endothelial denudation and damage to both intima and media.
	
	RBC-rich thrombus
	Platelet-rich thrombus
	Fibrin-rich thrombus

Acute Coronary Syndromes

POBA-induced changes in the plaques in acute coronary syndromes are essentially different from those in stable angina pectoris, due to the preexisting thrombus and ejected lipid pool debris.

Fig. 5 shows POBA-induced changes in the obstructed RCA in a patient with acute myocardial infarction. Angiographically, repeated balloon dilatation resulted in dilatation of the obstructed segment. However, obstruction of the posterior descending artery arising from the RCA (4PD) remained. Angioscopically, a red thrombus occupied the obstructed

Table 2
**IVUS Classification of POBA-Induced
Changes in the Culprit Plaques**

Minor changes
  Uneven surface
  Derrangement of plaque frame
Major changes
  1) Dissection
    Cleft (split), single or multiple within the fibrous cap
    extending to the lipid pool or extending to the media
    Cavity (echolucent space) formation in the plaque
    Intimal flap
    Separation of intima and media
  2) Bleeding and thrombus

segment before POBA. Repeated dilatation resulted in recanalization of the segment; however, a mural thrombus remained. In addition, a saddle thrombus was found at the bifurcation of 4PD and left ventricular branch. Since the thrombus contained crystals reflecting illumination, it may have detached from the obstructed segment and flown downstream to cause saddle thrombus. This thrombus became gradually smaller and finally disappeared during infusion of tPA (Fig. 6).

In our experience in a small number of patients with acute coronary syndromes due to occlusion with thrombus, residual thrombus at the POBA site was found in the majority of patients, and distal embolism was not infrequently observed (Table 3). This finding suggests the necessity of combined use of thrombolytic therapy and POBA.

Acute Occlusion and Its Predictors

Acute coronary artery occlusion after POBA continues to remain a serious complication, despite significant improvement in operator performance and technological advancements. It occurs in approximately 10% of patients. Its frequency is higher in patients with unstable angina, multivessel disease, and complex plaques.[4] Angioscopically, yellow plaque, disruption, and thrombus are predictors of acute occlusion.[5]

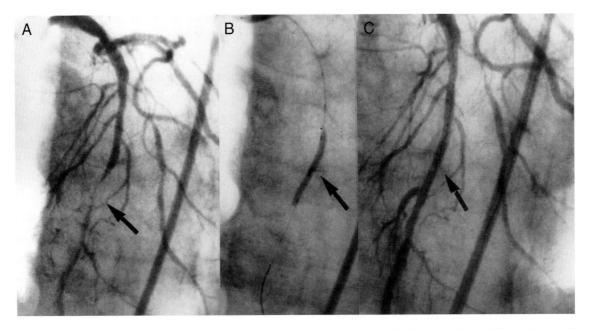

Fig. 1. M.N., 70-year-old female. Stable angina pectoris. Angiograms of the LAD before (**A**), during (**B**), and immediately after POBA. Arrows: target plaque.

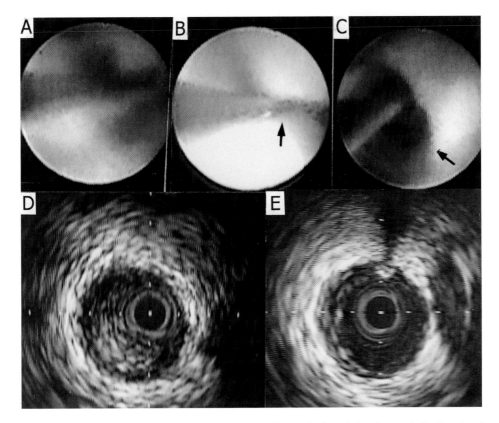

Fig. 2. The same patient as in Fig. 1. Angioscopic images of the plaque before (**A**), a large cleft after the first dilatation (arrow in **B**), and after repeated dilatation (**C**), and IVUS images before (**D**) and after repeated dilatation (**E**).

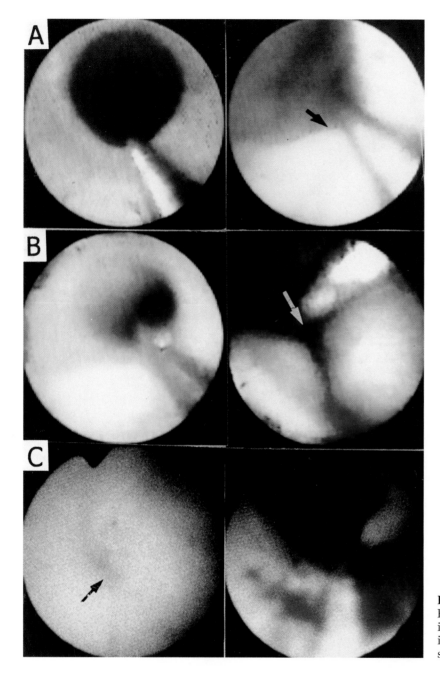

Fig. 3. Representative angioscopic images of POBA-induced plaque changes. **A:** POBA-induced tear of membranous plaque. **B:** cleft in the plaque. **C:** recanalization of an obstructive plaque.

Stable Angina Pectoris

Fig. 7 shows a concentric stenosis in the middle segment of the LAD. Angioscopically, a regular and white plaque was found in the stenotic segment. Angiographically, POBA resulted in dilatation but haziness remained. Haziness is attributable to the angioscopically demonstrated multiple intimal flaps and exposed yellow atheromatous tissues that occupied the lumen.

Fig. 8 shows representative angioscopic changes of acute occlusion with exposed calcium fragments, some with yellowish brown atheromatous tissue and some with reddish brown matter (probably a mixture of thrombus and atheromatous tissue, liquid or solid). In addition to occlusive changes in the targeted plaque, extensive dissection extending to nonstenotic segments occasionally occurs.

Fig. 9 shows a long dissection in the left circumflex coronary artery (LCx). By IVUS, the dissection ex-

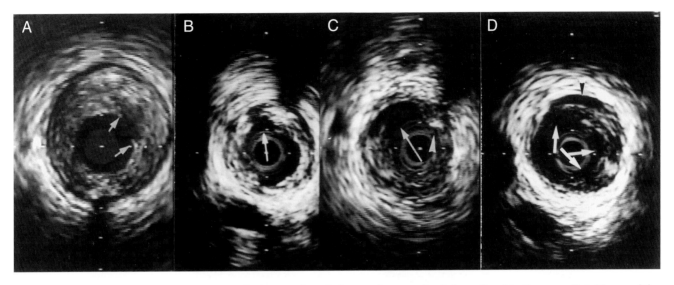

Fig. 4. Representative angioscopic images of POBA-induced plaque changes. **A:** cleft confined to the superficial layer of the intima (arrows). **B:** small cleft extending to the media (arrow). **C:** large cleft extending to the media (arrow). **D:** multiple clefts (arrows). Arrowheads in **C** and **D:** calcification and separation of intima and media, respectively.

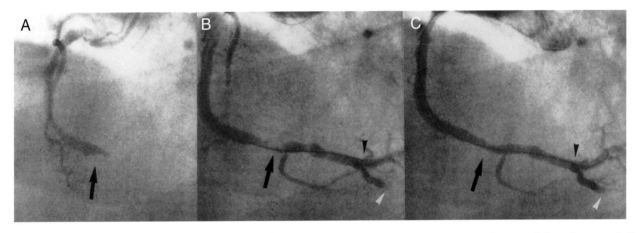

Fig. 5. K.H., 57-year-old male. Acute myocardial infarction. Before (**A**), initial (**B**), and repeated POBA (**C**) to obstructed distal segment of the RCA. Arrows: POBA site. Black arrows: bifurcation of 4PD and left ventricular branch. White arrows: obstructed 4PD.

tended from the proximal segment into its branches. Angioscopically, a thin and white intima was dissected and obstructed the lumen, indicating that dissection extended to the normal intima. The lumen was dilated during systole and collapsed during diastole.

Acute Coronary Syndromes

Angioscopic images of acute reocclusion following POBA in acute coronary syndromes (unstable angina and acute myocardial infarction) are different than those in stable angina due to the preexisting thrombus and atheromatous tissues in the lumen.

Fig. 10 shows angiographic and angioscopic changes induced by POBA in the proximal segment of the LAD in a patient with acute myocardial infarction. In this patient, POBA resulted in relief of chest pain and ST elevation. After a few minutes, however, chest pain and ST elevation reappeared. Angiography revealed a flap in the dilated segment that was

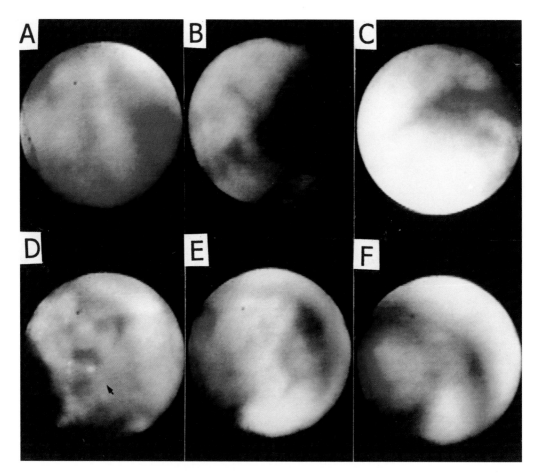

Fig. 6. The same patient as in Fig. 5. POBA site before (**A**), initial (**B**), and after repeated dilatation (**C**). Saddle thrombus at the bifurcation of 4PD and left ventricular branch before (**D**), 5 (**E**), and 10 minutes (**F**) after the beginning of selective tPA infusion into the artery. Arrow in **D:** crystals (cholesterol or calcium).

large and yellow with a red thrombus obstructing the lumen. The flap swung in synchrony to each cardiac beat and closed or opened the small residual lumen.

Likewise, acute reocclusion in acute coronary syndromes was due mainly to the mixture of atheromatous tissues and thrombus (Fig. 11). This angioscopic finding supports the concept that the predic-

Table 3
Angioscopic Changes in the Coronary Segments Occluded With Thrombus in Patients With Acute Coronary Syndromes Successfully Treated by POBA

	No. of Patients	Before POBA	After POBA
Occlusive thrombus	36	36	0
Mural thrombus			33
Distal thromboembolism			7

tors of acute reocclusion are yellow plaque, disruption, and thrombus.[5]

Acute Recoil

In addition to dissection and thrombosis, recoil is considered to be a major mechanism for restenosis or reocclusion that occurs several minutes or a few hours after POBA. In order to clarify the mechanisms for this phenomenon, we observed the plaques immediately after and 10 minutes after POBA was completed as shown in Fig. 12. A large intimal flap that was not observed immediately after was detached and obstructed the lumen after 10 minutes (Fig. 12A). In another patient, multiple flaps were compressed onto the wall immediately after POBA. Ten minutes later, however, they were separated from each other again and narrowed the lumen (Fig. 12B). These 2 changes are called "acute recoil." In a patient with acute coronary syndromes, a mural thrombus on fractured

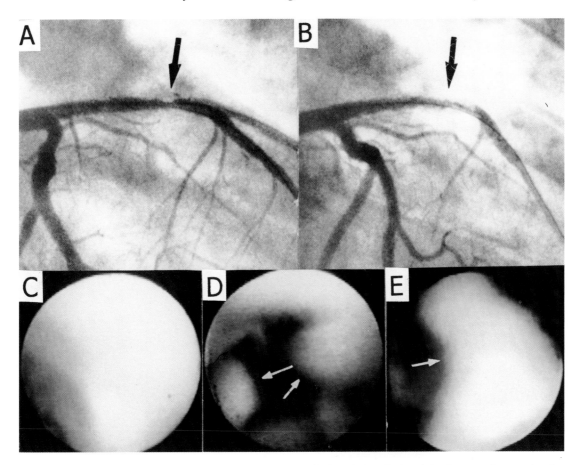

Fig. 7. S.I., 60-year-old male. Stable angina pectoris. Angiograms before (**A**) and after (**B**) POBA to the proximal segment of the LAD (arrows). **C:** regular and white plaque before POBA. **D:** intimal flaps in the proximal portion of the dilated segment (arrows). **E:** atheromatous mass behind the intimal flaps (arrow).

plaque was observed immediately after POBA. Ten minutes later, a glistening yellow plaque appeared. The plaque and its surroundings were amorphous and protruded into the lumen, suggesting swelling of the plaque (Fig. 12C). In a patient with acute coronary syndromes, a thrombus was compressed onto the wall immediately after POBA. Ten minutes later, however, the thrombus became cotton candy-like and obstructed the lumen, suggesting swelling of the thrombus. These findings suggest that not only elastic recoil but also swelling of atheroma and thrombus participate in acute restenosis and reocclusion after POBA.

POBA-Induced Unwanted Changes in the Coronary Segment Proximal to the Culprit Plaque

Angioscopic Changes

Coronary endothelial cells are very susceptible to mechanical stimuli. Therefore, balloon catheters and even soft-tipped guidewires, which are generally used for POBA, can easily cause damage to the proximal coronary segments, even by their simple passing, inappropriate pushing, inappropriate positioning, and/or dislocation of the balloon during dilatation.[2,6]

Fig. 13 shows representative examples of POBA-induced changes in the proximal segments: endothelial exfoliation, intimal flap, compression and bleeding, and uneven surface which was diffusely stained in blue with Evans blue, which selectively stains damaged endothelial cells (see Chapter 9). Thus, mechanically induced changes in the proximal segment were observed by conventional angioscopy in 63% of patients and in all by dye image angioscopy (Table 4).

Intravascular Ultrasonographic (IVUS) Changes

By IVUS, nonprotruded (lined) plaques are frequently observed in the angiographically non-

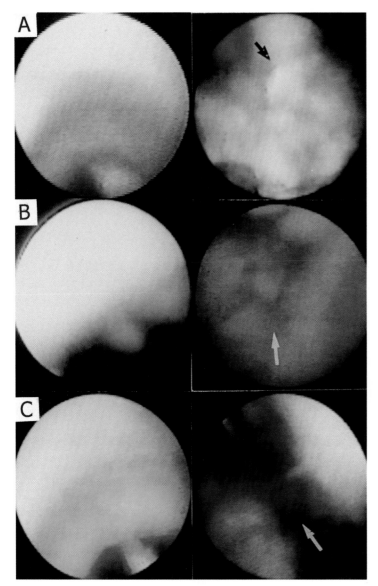

Fig. 8. Representative angioscopic images of acute occlusion. **Left:** before POBA. **Right:** after POBA. **A:** calcium crystals obstructing the lumen. **B:** yellowish brown amorphous atheromatous tissues obstructing the lumen. **C:** reddish brown material obstructing the lumen.

stenotic segments proximal to the plaques targeted for POBA. After POBA, linear low echoic spaces are not infrequently observed in these plaques. It is likely that inappropriate positioning of the balloon or its dislocation during dilatation directly deformed the plaque, or retrograde propagation of the fissure from the culprit plaque may have caused splitting of the frames in the proximal nonstenotic plaque (Fig. 14 and Table 4).

Changes in Chronic Stage

Changes 1 month or more after POBA are classified into those with restenosis and those without. The changes are different between stable angina pectoris and acute coronary syndromes.

Stable Angina Pectoris

Fig. 15A shows a cleft covered with endothelium observed 6 months after POBA. Likewise, such remnants of POBA-induced changes were observed in a small number of plaques at 6 months but not at 12 months (Table 5). Fig. 15B shows a dilated segment at 6 months after POBA. The luminal surface before POBA and immediately after POBA was yellow, but it was changed into white, resembling a coconut milk jelly-like surface 6 months later, probably due to neointima. In addition, the surface reflected illumination, exhibiting a glistening white surface. Irrespective of the color before POBA, the surface of the dilated segment glistened, reflecting illumination in the majority of plaques 6 to 12 months later (Table 5).

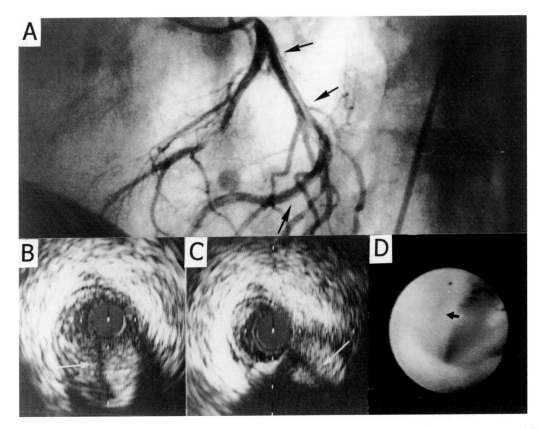

Fig. 9. K.K., 58-year-old female. POBA-induced long dissection in LCx (arrows in A) **B** and **C:** IVUS images of dissection in LCx and its branch, respectively. Arrows: exfoliated intima. **D:** angioscopic image of the exfoliated white intima (arrow).

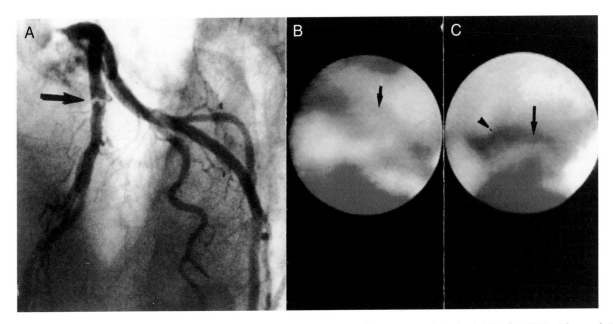

Fig. 10. K.I., 48-year-old male. Acute myocardial infarction. **A:** a large flap appeared in the LAD after POBA (arrow). **B:** a large yellow flap with red thrombus occluding the lumen during diastole. **C:** appearance of a residual lumen due to shift of the flap during systole. Arrows: flap. Arrowhead: residual lumen.

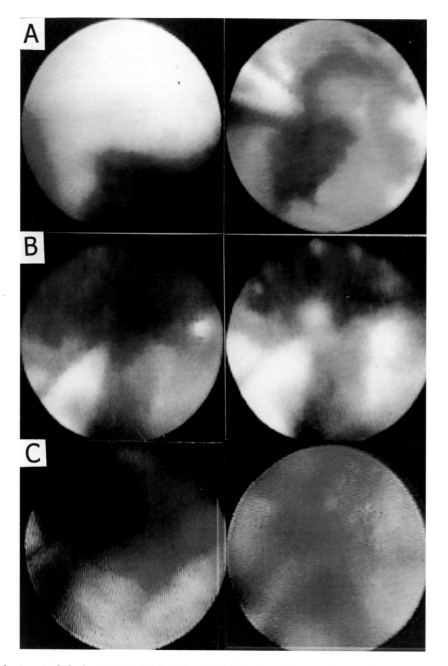

Fig. 11. Acute reocclusion. **Left:** before POBA. **Right:** after POBA. **A:** thrombus on disrupted glistening yellow plaque before and reocclusion with the mixture of atheromatous tissues and thrombus after. **B:** occlusion with the mixture of thrombus and atheromatous tissues before and reocclusion with the same mixture after. **C:** narrowing with thrombus on disrupted plaque before and occlusion with brown atheromatous tissues after.

Acute Coronary Syndromes

In patients with acute coronary syndromes, especially with acute myocardial infarction, yellow disrupted plaques with thrombus are frequently observed before and immediately after POBA. Four months later, however, they change into regular and coconut milk jelly-like white plaques in the majority of patients, probably due to cover of the exposed atheromatous tissues with the neointima (Table 5).

Restenosis and Its Predictors

Restenosis occurs in 30–60% of patients after POBA. Two major mechanisms are considered to participate in restenosis: intimal proliferation due to re-

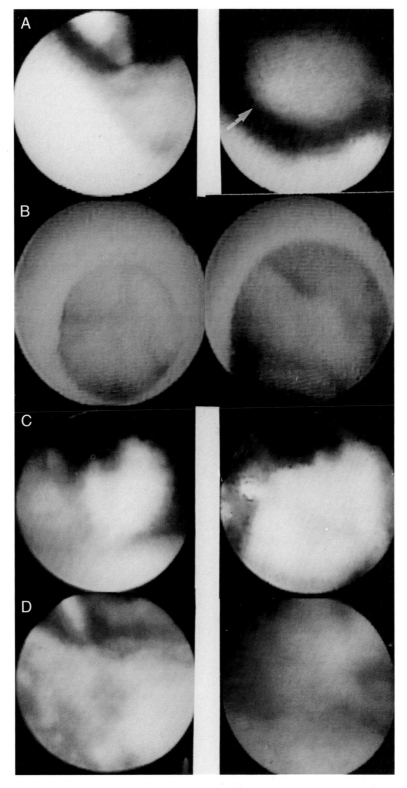

Fig. 12. Acute restenosis and reocclusion. **Left:** immediately after POBA. **Right:** 10 minutes after POBA. **A:** an intimal flap separated from the wall. **B:** multiple flaps separated from the wall. **C:** swelling of atheromatous tissues. **D:** swelling of thrombus.

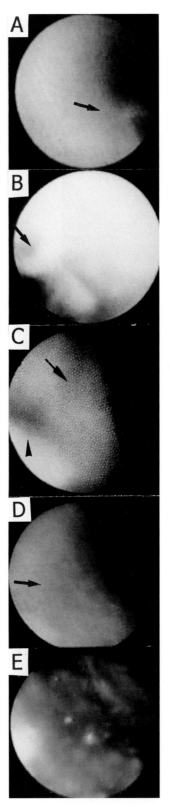

Fig. 13. POBA-induced changes in the segments proximal to the targeted plaque. **A:** endothelial exfoliation. **B:** intimal flap. **C:** compressed portion surrounded by bleeding. **D:** uneven surface. **E:** same portion as that in D, which was stained with Evans blue.

Table 4
POBA-Induced Changes in the Segments Proximal to the Culprit Plaques in Patients With Stable Angina Pectoris

	Before	*After POBA*
1) Angioscopy		
Total no. of segments	40	40
Stained with Evans blue	(−)	40
Uneven surface	0	8
Bleeding	0	11
Compression	0	3
Endothelial exfoliation	0	18
Flap	0	4
Dissection	0	5
Thrombus	0	6
2) IVUS		
No. of segments	0	20
Linear low echoic space		11
within the plaque		8
connecting to the lumen		3
Flaps		2
Dissection (cleft)		1

action of smooth muscle cells and platelets, and elastic recoil of overstretched atherosclerotic lesions.[7] Contraction of smooth muscle cells after recovery from stunning may also participate in restenosis.[8] Angioscopic predictors of restenosis were examined by several workers. Bauters observed that restenosis occurs more frequently in complex than in regular plaques.[9] Itoh noted that it occurs more frequently in white than in yellow plaques.[10] However, it is still controversial as to the angioscopic predictors of restenosis.

Development of dye or fluorescent angioscopy to differentiate substances such as myosin heavy chain isoforms of vascular smooth muscles[11] may be necessary for angioscopic prediction of restenosis.

Directional Coronary Atherectomy (DCA)

DCA is used mainly to remove eccentric plaques located in the proximal coronary segments. Figs. 16 and 17 show that a white plaque was smoothly debulked with resultant exposure of the remaining atheromatous tissues. Debulking was, however, insufficient by IVUS.

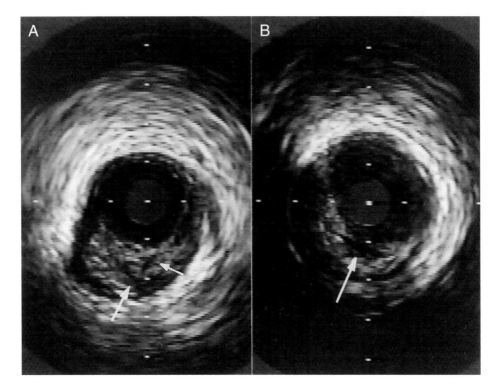

Fig. 14. IVUS changes in nontargeted proximal segments. **A:** multiple linear low echoic lines, indicating frame breakdown within a nonstenotic plaque. **B:** a linear low echoic space, indicating splitting within a nonstenotic plaque.

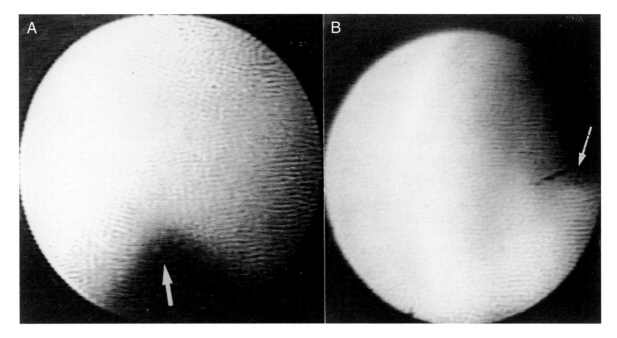

Fig. 15. Changes in POBA sites 6 months later. **A:** cleft covered with endothelium. **B:** coconut milk jelly-like surface.

Table 5
POBA-Induced Changes in the Culprit Plaques in Chronic Stage

	Before POBA	Immediately After POBA	1	4	6	12 months after
1) Stable angina pectoris						
No. of plaques	30	30	26	0	20	20
Cleft	0	27	4		3	0
Flap	0	21	2		0	0
White	18	7	12		16	15
Yellow or mosaic	9	23	14		4	5
Glistening yellow	3	0			0	
2) Acute coronary syndromes*						
No. of plaques	6	3				
Flap	5	0				
Thrombus	5	0				
White	0	2				
Yellow	5	1				

*Used with permission from ref. 13.

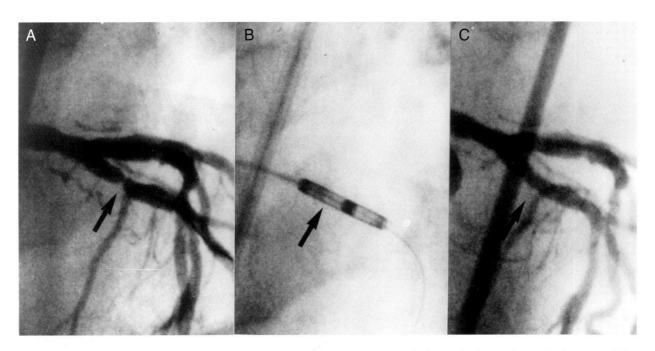

Fig. 16. R.U., 65-year-old male. Stable angina pectoris. Coronary angiograms before (**A**), during (**B**) and after DCA (**C**) to a segmental stenosis in the proximal segment of the LAD (arrows).

Stent Implantation

Angioscopic changes immediately after stent implantation depend on the changes induced by predilatation and the character of the preexisting thrombus. Therefore, the stent-induced changes in patients with acute coronary syndromes are different from those in patients with stable angina pectoris.[12–14]

Acute Changes

Stable Angina Pectoris

Fig. 18 shows angiographic changes in the stenotic middle segment of the LAD before and after predilatation by POBA, and after implantation of a MultiLink stent. Angioscopically, a regular and light

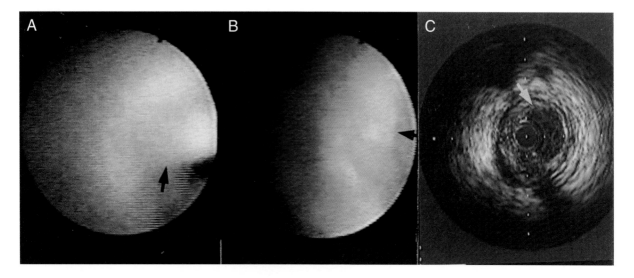

Fig. 17. The same patient as in Fig. 16. **A:** white plaque before directional coronary atherectomy (DCA) (arrow). **B:** exposed yellow atheromatous tissues after DCA. **C:** IVUS image of the same portion after DCA (arrow).

yellow plaque was found in the stenotic segment before. Predilatation by POBA caused a deep cleft in the plaque. The split plaque was compressed against the wall with the stent struts. However, thin mural thrombi were observed on the stent struts covering the dilated portion. Sufficient dilatation was confirmed by IVUS.

Immediately after stenting, protrusion of the wall through the space between the struts, white or yellow flaps, thrombus, and hemorrhage are frequently observed (Fig. 19; Table 6). When 2 or more stents are implanted in a series, they should be implanted in an overlapping fashion, unless the vascular wall between the 2 stents forms a bank (Fig. 19). This finding indicates the importance of overlapping one stent edge over the other.

Immediately after stenting, stent strut surface generally becomes like a frosty glass, irrespective of the stents implanted and despite the use of heparin and antiplatelet agents, as observed in animal experiments (see Chapter 9). In our study, the stent strut exhibiting such a change was stained in blue with Evans blue, indicating that fibrin networks were formed on them (Fig. 20).

Acute Coronary Syndromes

Angioscopic changes in the stented segments are more complex and dirty due to the preexisting thrombus and the debris from the lipid pool, the color of which is yellow or brown.

Fig. 21 shows angiographic and angioscopic images of the stent-implanted segment of the RCA in a patient with acute myocardial infarction. Before stenting, the proximal end of the obstructed portion was composed of yellow intimal flaps and reddish brown thrombi. Stent implantation successfully dilated the segment angiographically. Angioscopically, however, a considerable amount of reddish brown matter remained and the stent struts were buried in this matter. This matter is a mixture of thrombus and debris. Unlike patients with stable angina pectoris, protrusion of multiple atheromatous tissues into the lumen through the space between the struts was frequently observed. In addition, these tissues seemed to swell gradually (Fig. 22).

Angioscopically, thrombi remain in the majority of stent sites and flaps were also observed not infrequently (Tables 7 and 8). By IVUS, the echolucent spaces in the disrupted plaques disappear after stenting (Table 9).

Observation of Stent Edges and Side Branch Patency

Angioscopy is more accurate for observation of stent edge location and edge effects. Fig. 23A clearly shows that the proximal stent edge was appropriately dilated and caused no obvious damage to the vascular wall (no edge effects). Also, angioscopy is feasible for confirmation of side branch patency. Fig. 23B and

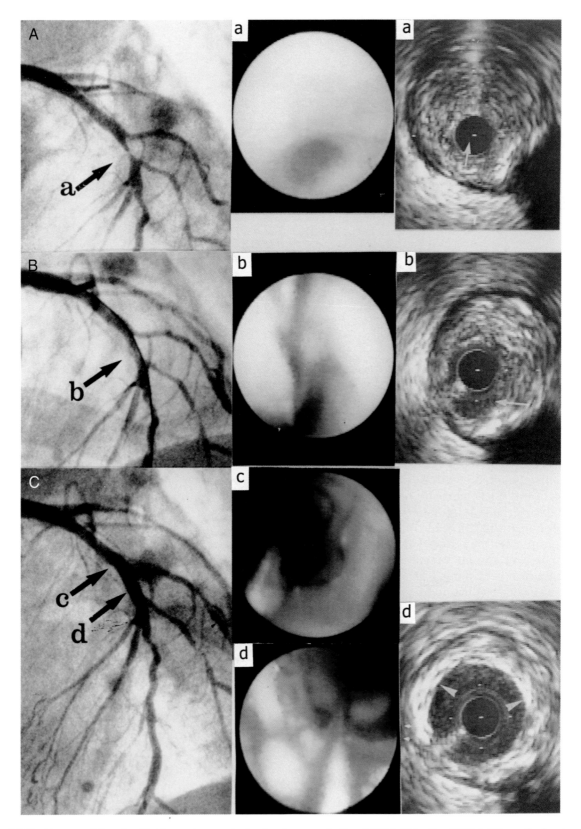

Fig. 18. M.K., 63-year-old male. Stable angina pectoris. Angiograms before POBA (**A**), after POBA (**B**), and after implantation of a MultiLink stent (**C**). Angioscopic images a, b, c, and d correspond to angiograms a, b, c, and d, respectively. IVUS images a, b, and d correspond to angiograms a, b, and d, respectively.

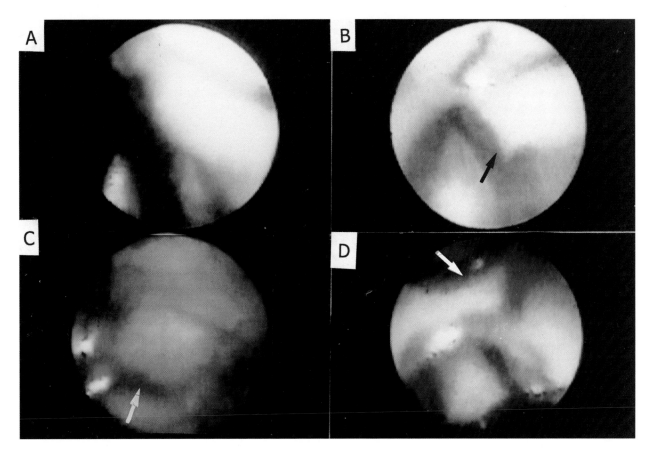

Fig. 19. Representative unwanted minor changes associated with stent implantation in patients with stable angina pectoris. **A:** protrusion of white wall between the stent struts into the lumen (arrow). **B:** a white intimal flap protruding into the lumen (arrow). **C:** a relatively large yellow intimal flap protruding into the lumen (arrow). **D:** bank formation between 2 stents (arrow).

Table 6
Angioscopic Follow-Up of Stented Coronary Segments in Patients With Stable Angina Pectoris

	Immediately After Stenting	*1*	*6 Months*
No. of plaques	23 (%)	20 (%)	15 (%)
Flap	6 (26)	1 (5)	0
Thrombus			
before Evans blue	14 (60)	7 (35)	2 (13)
after Evans blue	23 (100)		
Hemorrhage	13 (58)	2 (10)	0
White	11 (43)	13 (65)	11 (73)
Yellow or mosaic	12 (52)	7 (35)	4 (28)
Stent cover with endothelium			
Complete		15 (75)	14 (92)
Incomplete		3 (15)	1 (6)
Partial		2 (10)	0

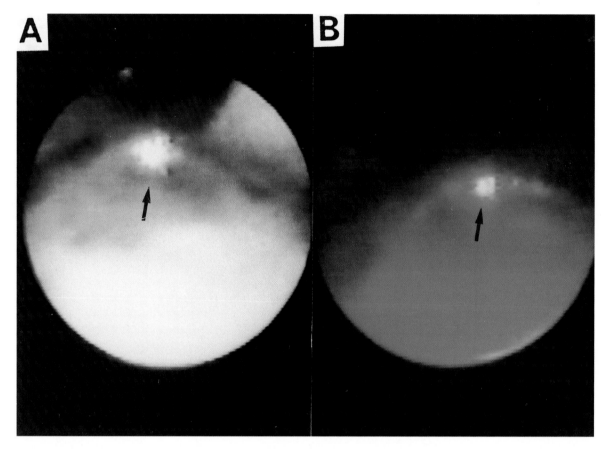

Fig. 20. Palmaz-Schatz stent. **A:** before Evans blue. The stent struts were covered with pink to whitish cotton candy-like matter. **B:** after Evans blue. The stent struts were stained in dark blue, indicating existence of fibrin.

C show existence of backflow from a side branch on which stent struts override, indicating its patency.

Acute and Subacute In-Stent Occlusion

Serious complications of stent implantations are acute and subacute occlusions. Fig. 24 shows angioscopic and IVUS images of acute occlusion occurring immediately after stenting. The proximal portion of the stent body was patent. However, the middle portion of the body was occluded with the mixture of fragmented atheromatous tissues and red thrombus. Identification of the substances occluding that portion was difficult by IVUS.

Subacute in-stent occlusion is referred to as "subacute thrombosis" (SAT). It occurs within a few days after stenting. In a patient with stable angina, a Gianturco-Roubin II coil stent was implanted into the proximal segment of the LAD. However, a flap remained in the stent (Fig. 25B). Three days later, an anginal attack and ST elevation in the electrocardiogram occurred despite the use of full doses of an-

tiplatelet agents. Angiography revealed hazy obstruction of the stented segment (Fig. 25C). Angioscopy revealed a pink and amorphous cotton candy-like thrombus obstructing the entire stent body (Fig. 26A). Thrombolysis failed to recanalize. Therefore, stent in-stent implantation using a Palmaz-Schatz stent was performed, with successful recanalization (Fig. 26C).

Time-Course Changes in the Stented Coronary Segments

Intimal flaps, thrombus, and hemorrhage that are observed immediately after stenting disappear in the majority of patients with stable angina pectoris (Table 6). In the majority of patients with acute coronary syndromes, however, in-stent thrombus remains in the majority of patients at 1 month (Fig. 27; Table 7). Although the reason is unclear, this fact indicates the necessity of enough anti-thrombotic therapy even after 1 month. Six months later, thrombus disappears in the majority of patients. The stent is

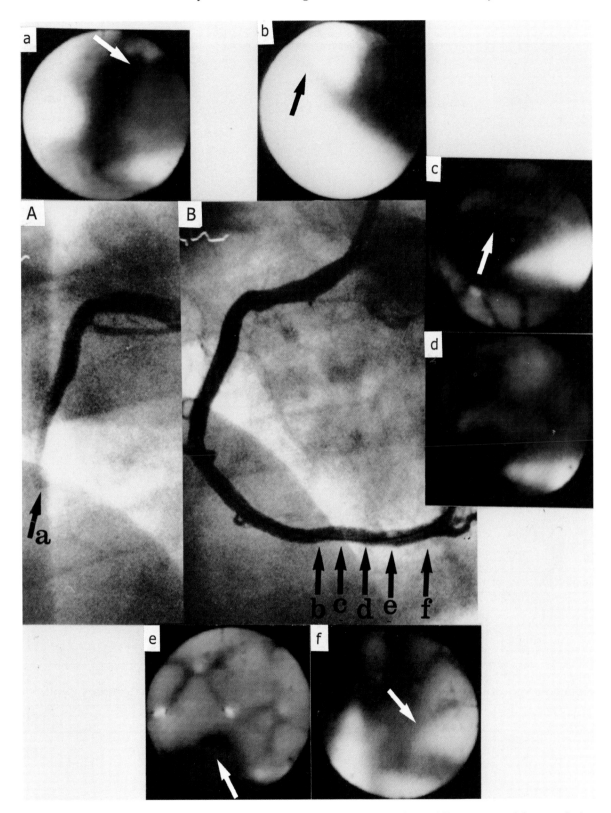

Fig. 21. A.T., 76-year-old male. Acute myocardial infarction. **A:** obstruction of the middle segment of the RCA before. **B:** after stent implantation to the distal segment of the RCA. Angioscopic images a to f correspond to those in angiograms, respectively. **a:** obstruction with red thrombus before stent implantation. **b:** white intimal flaps just proximal to the proximal stent edge (arrows). **c:** reddish brown matter occupying the lumen (arrow). **d:** closer observation of the matter. **e:** protrusion of white wall among the stent struts (arrow). **f:** yellow plaque at the distal stent edge (arrow).

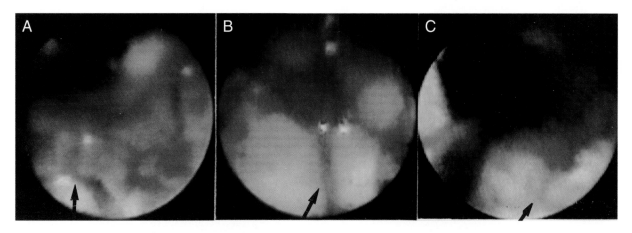

Fig. 22. Angioscopic changes immediately after stenting. **A:** relatively beautiful dilatation. **B:** protrusion of multiple atheromatous tissues between the struts into the lumen. **C:** swelling of the atheromatous tissues protruded between the struts into the lumen.

Table 7

Angioscopic Follow-Up of Stented Coronary Segments in Patients With Acute Coronary Syndromes

	Immediately After Stent	*1*	*3*	*6 Months*
1 Thrombus and flaps*				
No of plaques	30	19		12
Thrombus	21 (70%)	18 (95%)		0 (0%)
Flap	10 (33%)	2 (11%)		0 (0%)
2 Stent cover with endothelium				
No. of plaques	19*	21**		21**
Complete	4 (21%)	13 (61%)		18 (86%)
Incomplete	8 (42%)	5 (24%)		3 (14%)
Partial	7 (37%)	3 (14%)		0 (0%)

*Used with permission from ref. 12
**Used with permission from ref. 13.

Table 8

Angioscopic Follow-Up of Stented Coronary Segments in Patients with Acute Coronary Syndromes

	Immediately After Stenting	*2 Weeks*	*4 Months*
1. Hemorrhage			
No. of plaques	10	6	6
Hemorrhage	8 (80%)	4 (66%)	0 (0%)
2. Color of plaques**			
No. of plaques	18	16	8
Yellow	16 (88%)	14 (88%)	2 (25%)
White	2 (11%)	2 (12%)	6 (75%)

**Used with permission from ref. 14.

Table 9
Follow-Up of Stented Coronary Segments by IVUS

	Before POBA	After POBA	After Stent	2 Weeks	5 Months
No. of plaques	24	18	14	14	14
Tear	12 (50%)	10 (55%)	0 (0%)	0 (0%)	0 (0%)
Echolucent space in plaque	12 (50%)	12 (66%)	2 (14%)	1 (7%)	0 (0%)
Echolucent space communicated with lumen	8 (33%)	6 (33%)	0 (0%)	0 (0%)	0 (0%)

Used with permission from ref. 14.

covered with neointima in the majority of patients (Figs. 28, 29; Tables 6, 8).

Surface color of stented coronary segments changes into white in the majority of patients, due to stent coverage with neointima (Tables 6, 8). In a small number of patients, the luminal surface of the stented portion is yellow, probably due to deposition of beta-carotene or lipids into the neointima, or due to cover of residual atheromatous tissues with neointima (Fig. 28).

By IVUS, abnormal changes observed during stent implantation disappear before 6 months (Table 9).

Stent Cover with Endothelium

Stent struts remain uncovered with neointima even 6 months after stenting in a small number of patients (Tables 6, 7). Fig. 30 shows a patient in whom the stent struts in the distal portion remained uncovered with neointima even 6 months after stenting. The reason for it is not known. In addition to reduced potency of division of the neighboring endothelial cells and a lack of circulating progenitor cells, long-lasting thrombosis on the struts may act against endothelial cell migration and growth on the struts.

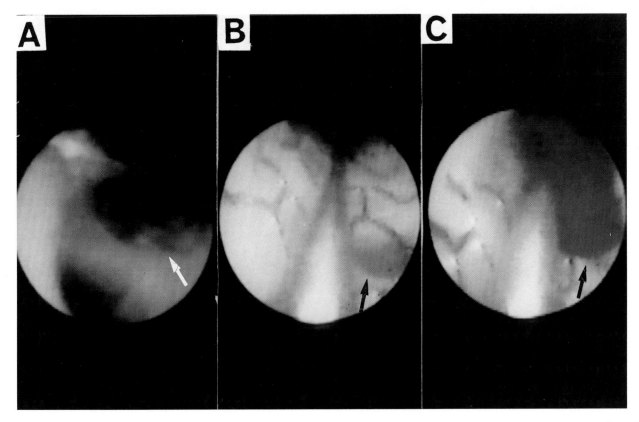

Fig. 23. A: proximal stent edge located just distal to a side branch ostium (arrow). **B:** a side branch ostium during diastole (arrow). **C:** backflow of blood from the side branch during systole (arrow).

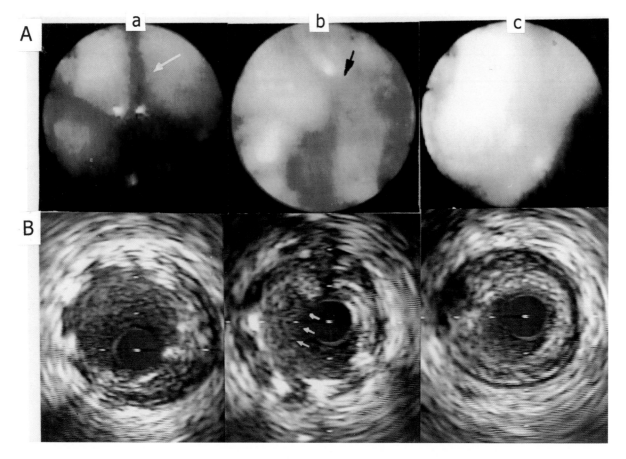

Fig. 24. C.K., 66-year-old male. Unstable angina pectoris. In-stent acute occlusion immediately after Palmaz-Schatz stent implantation to the middle segment of the RCA. Aa and Ba: proximal portion of the stent body. Ab and Bb: occlusion with the mixture of thrombus and atheromatous tissues in the middle portion of the stent body. Ac and Bc: the segment distal to the stent.

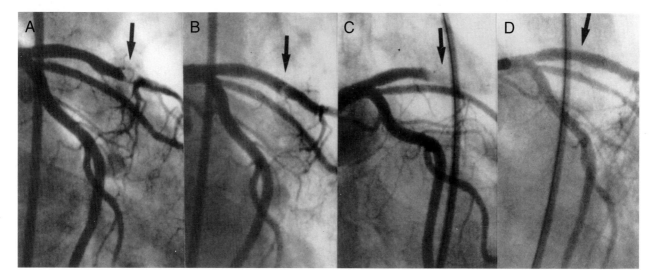

Fig. 25. M.Y., 73-year-old male. Stable angina pectoris. Angiograms before (**A**), immediately after stenting (**B**), subacute thrombosis (**C**), and after stent in-stent implantation (**D**).

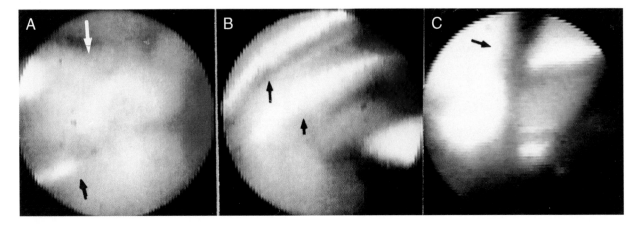

Fig. 26. The same patient as in Fig. 25. Angioscopic images before (**A**) and after thrombolytic therapy with tPA (**B**), and after stent in-stent implantation (**C**).

Function of Endothelial Cells Covering the Stent Struts

Damaged endothelial cells have strong affinity to fibrin. Therefore, if the new endothelial cells covering the stent struts are damaged, they may become a focus of thrombosis. Therefore, it is important to clarify whether the endothelial cells covering the stent struts are functioning normally. Fig. 31 shows 3 examples of apparently intact endothelial cells covering the struts observed by conventional angioscopy 6 months after stenting. The endothelial cells were stained with Evans blue in 2 of them, indicating that they are damaged by unknown mechanisms. Deformation and/or dislocation of the struts caused by cardiac motion may have caused endothelial cell damage. If so, use of stents with the same elasticity as the vascular wall should be taken into consideration.

In-Stent Restenosis

As in the case of other interventional therapies, restenosis also occurs in or at the edges of the implanted stent (in-stent restenosis). It occurs in 6% to 50% of stent procedures and within 6 months. Angiographically, in-stent restenosis is classified as diffuse or focal (Fig. 32). Diffuse restenosis occurs more frequently than focal restenosis (70–80% vs. 20–30%). The predictors for diffuse restenosis are long lesion, smaller vessel (internal diameter <2.8 mm), stenting without debulking, and high pressure balloon inflation, and the predictor for focal restenosis is diabetes mellitus.[15]

Fig. 33 shows coronary angiographic and angioscopic images of diffuse in-stent restenosis observed at 6 months after implantation of a Wiktor stent into the proximal to middle segment of the LAD in a patient with stable angina pectoris. Angioscopically, the luminal surface was diffusely bluish white and resembled coconut milk jelly due to intimal hyperplasia. The surface was uneven due to regional differences in neointimal hyperplasia. Stent struts were seen through where hyperplasia was mild. A coconut milk jelly-like luminal surface is a typical angioscopic change of intimal hyperplasia as in the case of POBA-induced restenosis. However, surface color does not necessarily exhibit such a white color. Fig. 34 shows a diffusely light yellow luminal surface from the restenotic proximal stent edge to the distal edge, probably due to lipid deposition into the hyperplasied intima.

By IVUS, there are 2 distinctly different types of restenosis: high echoic and low echoic. The surface color is bluish white in the majority of high echoic restenotic portions and yellow to brown in the majority of low echoic restenotic portions (Fig. 35). The underlying mechanism(s) for this difference is unclear, but there are the possibilities that intimal hyperplasia alone occurred in the former, and lipid deposition occurred mainly in the hyperplasied intima, or intimal hyperplasia occurred in the residual or recoiled atheromatous tissues.

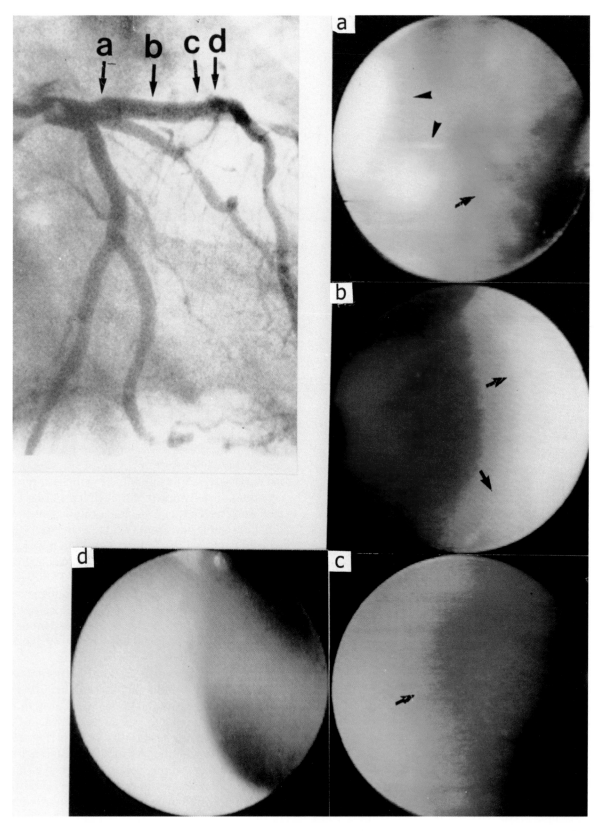

Fig. 27. A.K., 60-year-old male. Acute myocardial infarction. One month after direct stenting to the proximal segment of the LAD. Angioscopic images **a** to **d** correspond to those in angiograms, respectively. Arrow in a: thrombus. Arrowheads in a: glistening yellow flaps. Arrows in b: stent struts seen through the neointima. Arrow in c: thrombus.

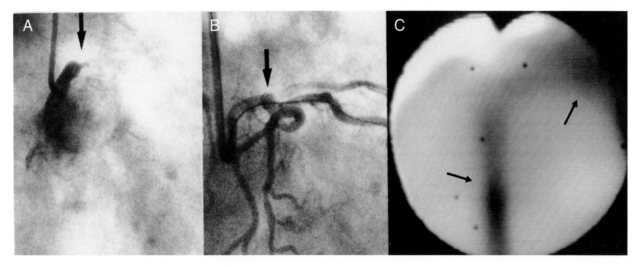

Fig. 28. S.S., 57-year-old male. Stable angina pectoris due to left main trunk stenosis. **A:** before stenting. **B:** after stenting. Angioscopic image of the stent site 6 months later. **C:** stent struts were seen through yellow neointima.

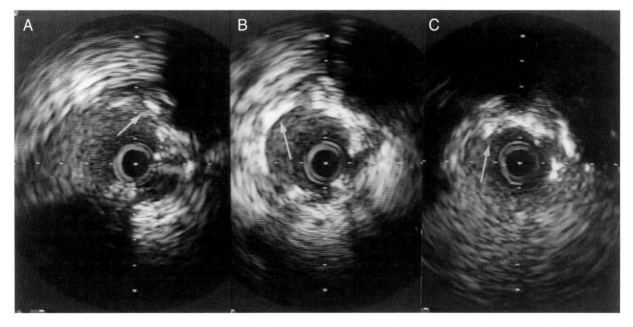

Fig. 29. The same patient as in Fig. 28. Location of the stent struts identified by IVUS. **A:** distal edge at the bifurcation of the LAD and LCx. **B:** stent body in the left main trunk. **C:** proximal edge protruded into the aorta.

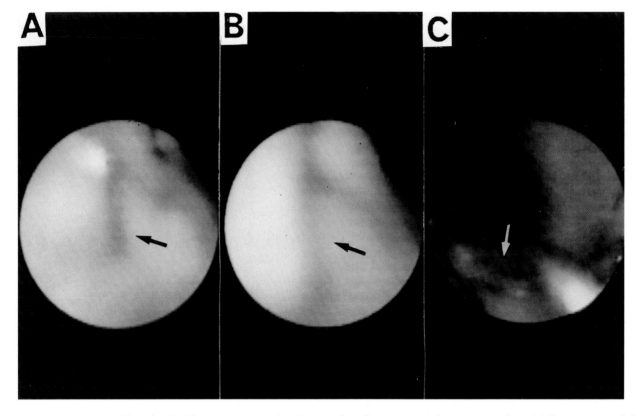

Fig. 30. S.H., 61-year-old male. Stable angina pectoris. Six months after stent implantation to the middle segment of the RCA. Stent struts covered with neointima in the proximal (**A**) and middle (**B**) portions, and those uncovered in the distal portion (arrow in C).

Cutting Balloon

A cutting balloon is frequently used for treatment of restenosis. Figs. 36 and 37 show the incised portion of an in-stent restenosis. In this patient with acute myocardial infarction, a MultiLink stent was successfully implanted into the LAD. However, in-stent restenosis was found 6 months later. The stenotic portion was successfully dilated by a cutting balloon. The incised portion was clearly demonstrated by both angioscopy and IVUS.

Angioscope-Guided Intracoronary Thrombolysis

Fig. 38 shows a segmental stenosis in the proximal segment of the LAD in a patient with unstable angina pectoris. Angioscopy revealed a white thrombus in the stenotic segment. tPA was selectively infused into the artery and the thrombus disappeared angioscopically; angiographic stenosis also disap-

peared 3 minutes after the beginning of infusion. Likewise, time-course changes in the thrombus were observed in 8 patients with acute coronary syndromes. The majority of mixed thrombi became white and then disappeared within 9 minutes (Table 10). It is likely that the red blood cells detached from the surface of the thrombus due to lysis of the fibrin network, the fibrin and platelet core was exposed, and then the exposed core was lysed to smaller ones and flowed downstream as was demonstrated in animal experiments (see Chapter 9).

Thrombus Aspiration

A large or long thrombus is frequently resistant to conventional interventions such as POBA, stent, or thrombolysis. Figs. 39 and 40 show obstruction of the distal segment of the RCA with red thrombus in a patient with acute myocardial infarction. Although the thrombus became smaller, sufficient recanalization was not attained. Therefore, the thrombus was aspirated using a 5 F catheter. This method is effective in selected patients.

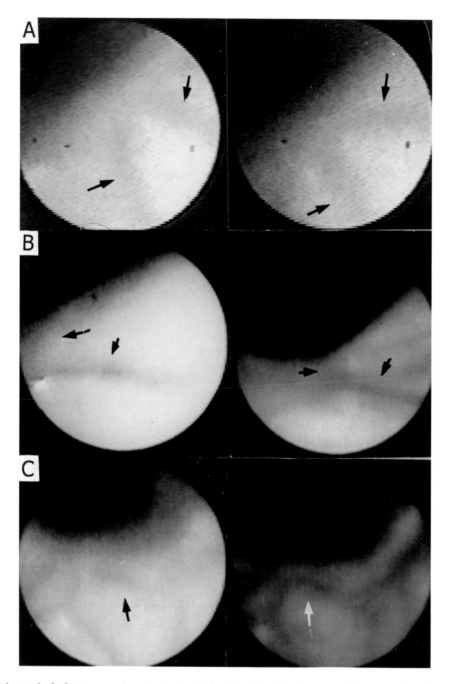

Fig. 31. Damage of the endothelium covering stent struts identified by dye image angioscopy using Evans blue. **Left:** before Evans blue. **Right:** after Evans blue. Endothelium covering the stent struts not stained (**A**); staining was confined to the endothelium on the struts (**B**); and not only the endothelium on the struts but also other portions were stained diffusely (**C**). Arrows: endothelium covering the stent struts.

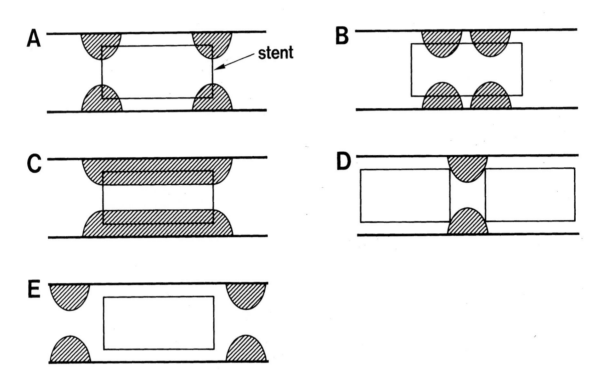

Fig. 32. Schematic representation of in-stent restenosis. Used with permission from ref. 15 and partially modified.

Table 10

Time-Course Changes in Coronary Thrombus During PTCR with tPA in Patients With Acute Coronary Syndromes

Thrombus Color	Before	3	6	9 Min After
Red	1	0	0	0
White	1	2	1	0
Mixed	7	5	3	1
Disappeared		1	4	7

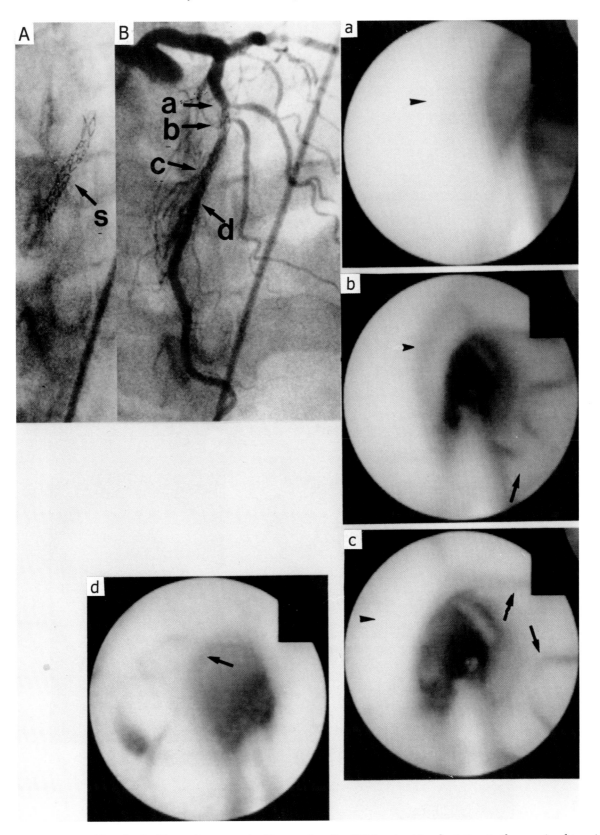

Fig. 33. A.Y., 67-year-old male. Stable angina pectoris. Six months after Wiktor stent implantation to the proximal to middle segment of the LAD. **A:** stent. **B:** angiogram showing in-stent restenosis. Angioscopic images **a** to **d** correspond to those in B, respectively. Arrows in angioscopic images: stent struts seen through the neointima. Arrowheads: neointima at the site of restenosis.

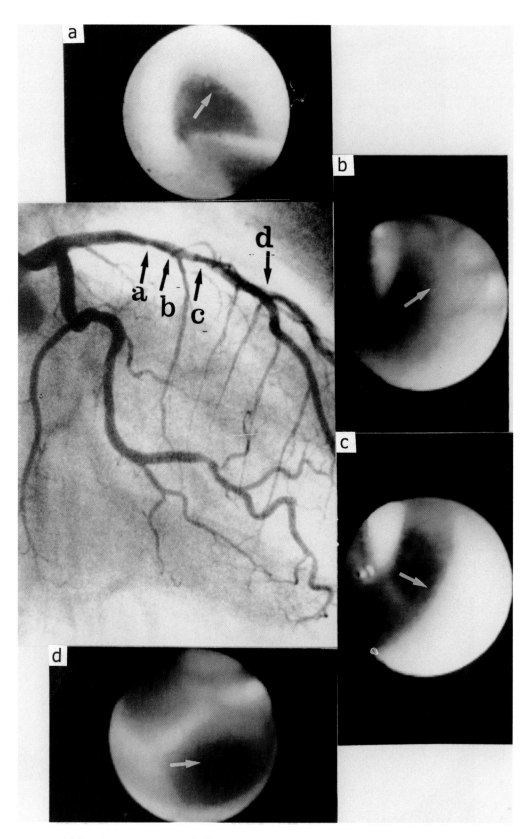

Fig. 34. A.Y., 70-year-old female. Acute myocardial infarction. Six months after stent implantation to the proximal segment of the LAD. Angioscopic images **a** to **d** correspond to those in angiogram. Arrow in a: restenosis at the proximal stent edge. Arrow in b: stent struts. Arrow in c: restenosis at the distal stent edge. Arrow in d: side branch just distal to c.

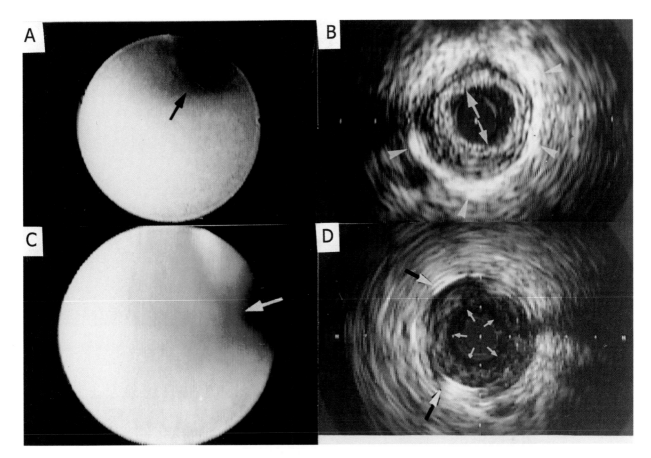

Fig. 35. Representative IVUS images of in-stent restenosis and their corresponding angioscopic images. **A:** white plaque. **B:** hard plaque that corresponds to A. **C:** yellow plaque. **D:** soft plaque that corresponds to C.

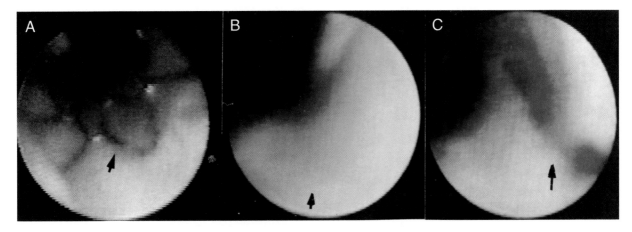

Fig. 36. K.M, 70-year-old male. Acute myocardial infarction. Angioscopic images immediately after stent implantation, 6 months after (**B**) and immediately after cutting by a cutting balloon (**C**). Arrow in A: stent strut. Arrow in B: stenotic portion. C: incised portion.

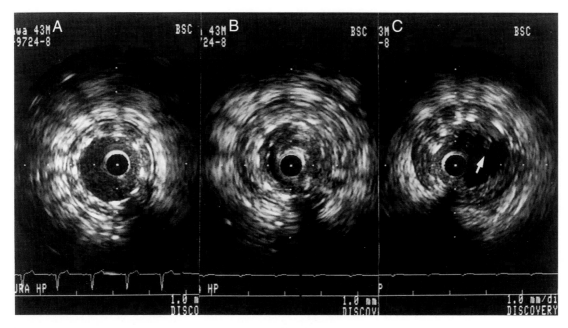

Fig. 37. The same patient as in Fig. 36. IVUS images of immediately after stenting (**A**), restenosis after 6 months (**B**), and immediately after dilatation by a cutting balloon (**C**).

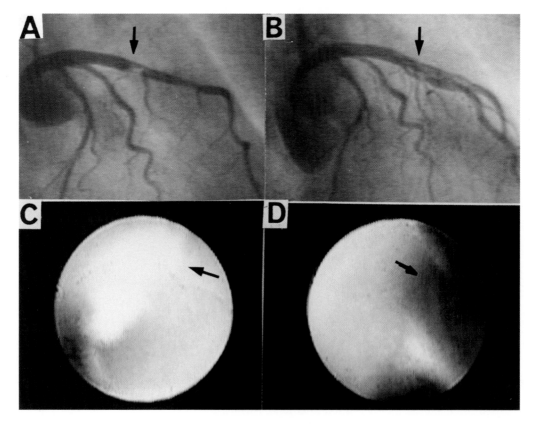

Fig. 38. N.T., 61-year-old male. Unstable angina pectoris. Coronary angiograms before (**A**) and 3 minutes after the beginning of tPA infusion (**B**). Angiograms before (**C**) and 3 minutes after the beginning of tPA infusion (**D**). Arrow in A: stenotic segment. Arrow in C: white thrombus. Plaque disruption was not detected by conventional angioscopy in this patient.

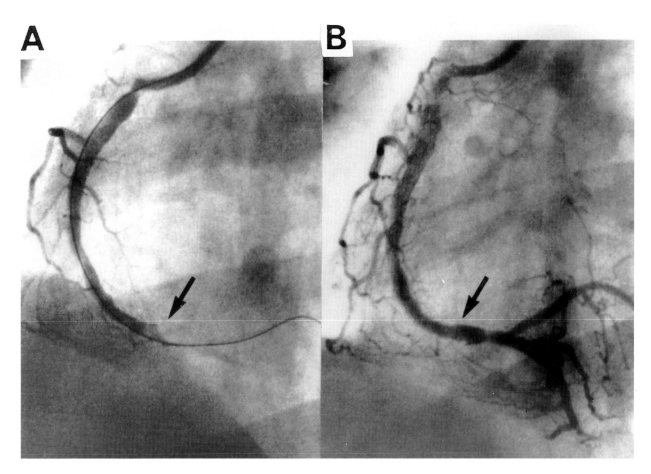

Fig. 39. K.I., 60-year-old male. Acute myocardial infarction. Coronary angiograms before (**A**) and after thrombus aspiration (**B**).

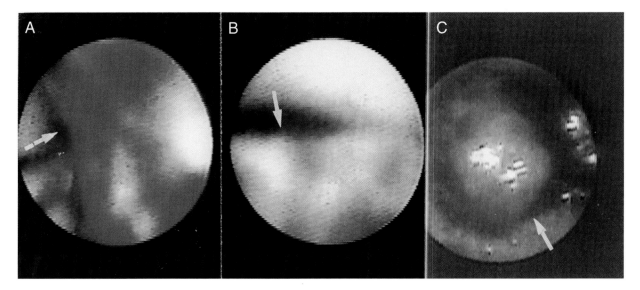

Fig. 40. The same patient as in Fig. 39. **A:** red thrombus before thrombolysis. **B:** mixed thrombus after thrombolysis. **C:** aspirated thrombus.

Coronary Angioscopy for Decision-Making of Additional Interventions

Coronary angiography is very weak in detecting intimal flaps and dissections and in differenti-

ation of thrombus from atherosclerotic plaque. Coronary angioscopy is feasible for detecting intimal flaps and dissections and for differentiation of thrombus from plaque. Therefore, we use angioscopy for decision-making of additional interventions (Table 11).

Table 11
Coronary Angioscopy for Decision-Making of Additional Interventions in Patients With Acute Coronary Syndromes

	Post-POBA		Decision of		Post-Stent	
	CAG	Angioscopy	Stent	Thrombolysis	CAG	Angioscopy
No. of patients	21	21			21	21
Flap	5	15	10		0	6
Dissection	0	2	1		0	0
Thrombus	3	11		5	0	9

References

1. Uchida Y, Masuo M, Tomaru T, et al: Fiberoptic observation of the luminal changes associated with transluminal coronary angioplasty. Circulation 58(Suppl):I-210, 1985.
2. Uchida Y, Hasegawa K, Kawamura K, et al: Angioscopic observation of coronary luminal changes induced by percutaneous transluminal coronary angioplasty. Am Heart J 117:1153–1155, 1989.
3. Ip JH, Fuster V, Badimon L: Syndromes of accelerated atherosclerosis: Role of vascular injury and smooth muscle cell proliferation. J Am Coll Cardiol 15:1667–1687, 1990.
4. de Feyter PJ, van den Brand M, Jaarman G, et al: Acute coronary artery occlusion during and after percutaneous transluminal coronary angioplasty. Circulation 83:927–936, 1991.
5. Waxman S, Sassouer MA, Mittleman MA, et al: Angioscopic predictors of early adverse outcome in patients with unstable angina and non-Q wave myocardial infarction. Circulation 93:2106–2116, 1996.
6. Uchida Y: Percutaneous coronary angioscopy. Jpn Heart J 33:271–294, 1992.
7. Waller BF, Pinkerton CA, Orr CM, et al: Restenosis 1 to 24 months after clinically successful coronary balloon angioplasty. J Am Coll Cardiol 17:58B-70B, 1991.
8. Mints GS, Pompa JJ, Pichard AD: Arterial remodeling after coronary angioplasty: A serial intravascular ultrasound study. Circulation 94:35–43, 1996.
9. Bauters C, Lablanche JM, McFadden EP: Relation of coronary angioscopic findings at coronary angioplasty to angiographic restenosis. Circulation 92:2473–2479, 1995.
10. Itoh A, Miyazaki S, Nonogi H, et al: Circulation 91:1389–1396, 1995.
11. Simons M, Leclerc G, Safian RD, et al: Relation between activated smooth muscle cells in coronary artery lesions and restenosis after atherectomy. N Engl J Med 328:608–613, 1992.
12. Fujimori Y, Morio H, Terasawa K, et al: Angioscopic follow-up study on stented plaques in acute myocardial infarction. Proceedings of the 13th Meeting of Cardioangioscopy and Laser Cardioangioscopy, p 28, 1999 (in Japanese).
13. Tsukahara R, Hou M, Muramatsu T: Characteristics of coronary plaques culprit for acute myocardial infarction in chronic stage. Coronary 15:145–150, 1998 (in Japanese).
14. Tsukahara R, Muramatsu T, Hou M, et al: Angioscopic and ultrasonographic follow-up study on the efficacy of direct stent in acute myocardial infarction. J Jpn Coll Angiol 39:17–22, 1999.
15. Kini A, Marmur JD, Dargas G, et al: Angiographic patterns of in-stent restenosis and implications of subsequent revascularization. Cathet Cardiovasc Interven 49:23–29, 2000.

Chapter 15

Coronary Bypass Grafts

Saphenous Vein Grafts

Saphenous vein grafts (SVGs) are observed during[1] and after operation by angioscopy and IVUS.[2,3] Fig. 1A shows angiograms of SVGs to the left anterior descending artery 1 month after grafting. Angioscopically, the anastomosed site to native artery was smoothly covered with endothelium (Fig. 2). Fig. 3 shows yellow plaques and neointima observed 1 year after grafting. These changes were not identified by angiography. IVUS is also feasible for observation of the changes in the SVG itself and in the anastomosed site to native artery (Figs. 4, 5).

Angioscopy is feasible for evaluation of interventional therapies of SVG obstruction. Fig. 6 shows a massive thrombus obstructing the entire SVG anastomosed to the LAD. The thrombus color was not uniform; it was fresh red, dark red, or brown, showing fresh and old thrombi in combination, indicating recurrent thrombosis. Angioscope-guided thrombolytic therapy with tPA resulted in successful recanalization by angiography. Angioscopically, however, massive mural thrombi remained (Fig. 7).

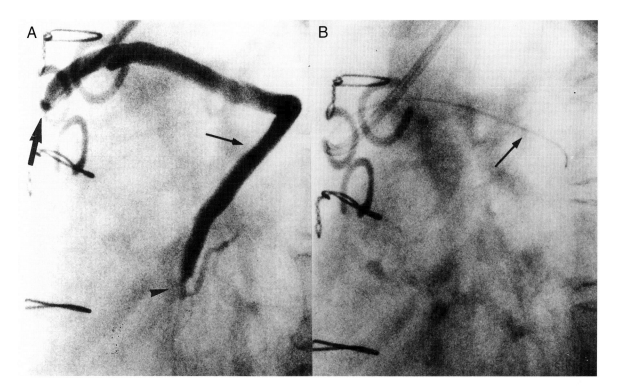

Fig. 1. N.R., 61-year-old male. Stable angina pectoris. One month after SVG to the LAD. **A:** angiogram of the graft (arrow). **B:** fiberscope introduced into the graft (arrow).

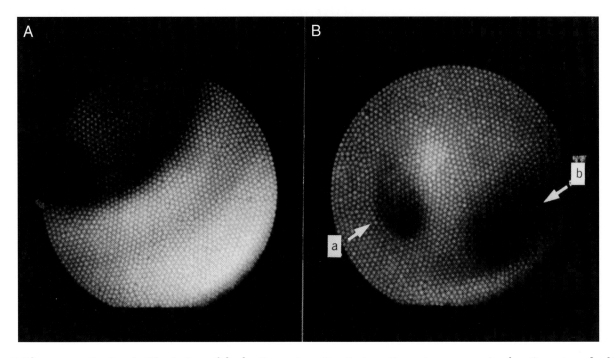

Fig. 2. The same patient as in Fig. 1. **A:** graft body. **B:** anastomotic site to native artery. **a:** proximal native artery. **b:** distal native artery.

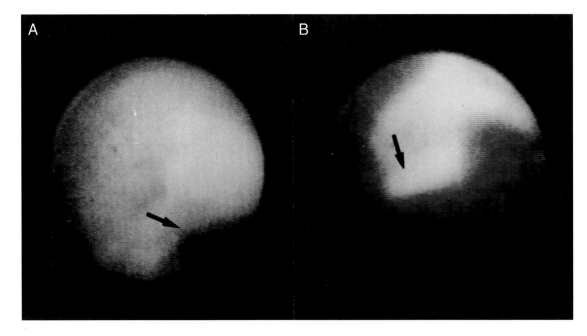

Fig. 3. K.K., 69-year-old male. Stable angina pectoris. One year after SVG to the LAD. **A:** yellow plaque in the graft. **B:** white neointima and red mural thrombus.

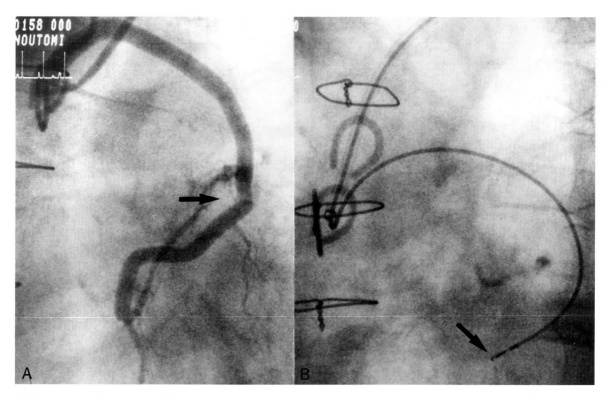

Fig. 4. I.U., 55-year-old male. Stable angina pectoris. One month after bridge grafting to the LAD and the first diagonal branch. **A:** angiogram of SVG showing a narrowing at the bridge anastomosis to the first diagonal branch (arrow). **B:** IVUS probe inserted into the graft (arrow).

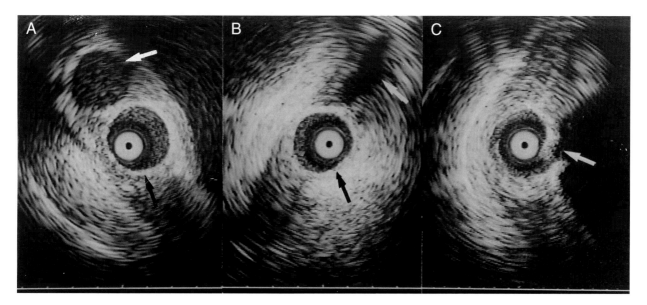

Fig. 5. The same patient as in Fig. 4. IVUS images of SVG 1 month after grafting. **A:** graft body. White arrow: LAD. Black arrow: graft body. **B:** anastomotic site to the first diagonal branch. White arrow: the first diagonal branch. Black arrow: graft. **C:** kinking of graft (arrow), which corresponds to narrowing in Fig. 4A.

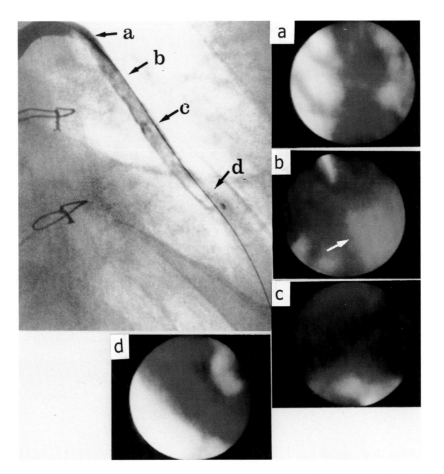

Fig. 6. A.I., 70-year-old male. One year after SVG to the LAD. Total occlusion of the SVG with thrombus. Angioscopic images a to d correspond to those in angiogram. Arrow in c: brown thrombus.

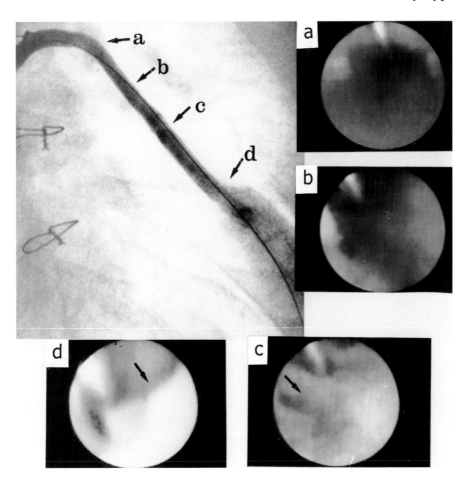

Fig. 7. The same patient as in Fig. 6. Recanalization after thrombolysis. Angioscopic images a to d correspond to those in angiogram, respectively.

References

1. Sanborn TA, Rygaard JA, Westbrook BM, Lazar HL, McCormick JR, et al: Intraoperative angioscopy of saphenous vein and coronary arteries. J Thoracic Cardiovasc Surg 9:339–341, 1986.
2. Uchida Y: Coronary angioscopy. Jpn Heart J 33: 271–294, 1992.
3. Annex BH, Ajiuni SC, Larkin TJ, et al: Angioscopic guided interventions in a saphenous vein bypass graft. Cathet Cardiovasc Interven 31:330–333, 1994.

Chapter 16

Prediction of Acute Coronary Syndromes by Coronary Angioscopy

It is still not predictable in whom, when, where, and under what conditions acute coronary syndromes (unstable angina pectoris and acute myocardial infarction) will occur. If they become predictable, the great burden they now place on humans may be minimized. Because of histological study using postmortem coronary specimens and clinical application of coronary angioscopy and intravascular ultrasound, considerable knowledge has been accumulated on plaque morphology and its clinical implications.

Angioscopically, coronary atherosclerotic plaques are classified, based on their surface appearance, into regular and complex plaques. The former plaques are further classified by color as white, light yellow, nonglistening yellow, and glistening yellow. Studies of the relationships between plaque color and histological changes in vitro revealed that a glistening yellow plaque is one major vulnerable plaque.[1]

To pinpoint the link between plaque appearance and acute coronary syndromes, we performed a 12-month prospective follow-up study in 157 patients with stable angina pectoris in whom regular coronary plaques alone were observed by percutaneous coronary angioscopy. Acute coronary syndromes occurred more frequently in patients with yellow plaques than in those with white plaques. Moreover, the syndromes occurred more frequently and in a shorter period of time in patients with glistening yellow plaques than in those with nonglistening yellow plaques (Table 1, Fig. 1). Thrombus arising from the disrupted identical plaques was confirmed by angioscopy as the culprit lesion of the syndromes (Figs. 2–5). Our results suggest that acute coronary syndromes occur frequently and in a short period of time in patients with glistening yellow coronary plaques. Further double-blind follow-up studies should be carried out to confirm this result. In the near future, based on angioscopic plaque characteristics, prophylactic modalities of these fatal syndromes may be established.

Table 1
Relationships Between Angioscopic Characteristics of the Coronary Plaques and the Clinical Outcome

Plaque	No. of Patients	No. of Plaques	Acute Coronary Syndromes			% Incidence	
			UA	AMI	Total	Patients	Plaque
White	118	182	1	3	4	3.3	2.1
Yellow	39	48	2	7	11	28.2	22.8
Yellow							
nonglistening	26	34	0	2	2	7.6	5.9
glistening	13	14	2	7	9	68.4	64.2

UA: unstable angina. AMI: acute myocardial infarction.

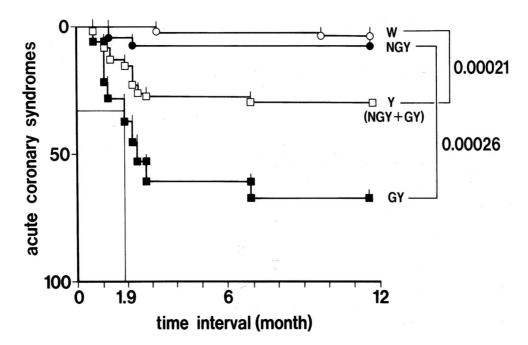

Fig. 1. Relationships between plaque color and occurrence of acute coronary syndromes. W: white plaque group. NGY: nonglistening yellow plaque group. GY: glistening yellow plaque group.

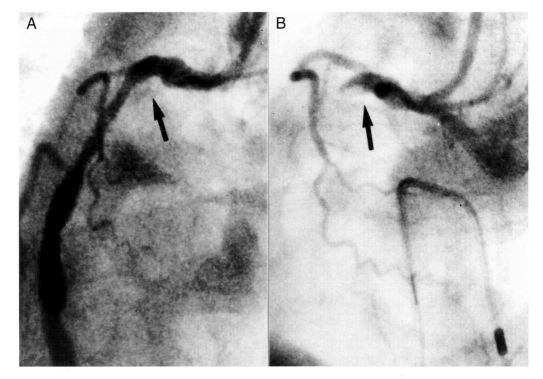

Fig. 2. M.R., 60-year-old male. **A:** angiogram before acute myocardial infarction showing a nonsignificant stenosis in the proximal segment of the RCA (arrow). **B:** total occlusion 3 hours after the onset of attack. Arrow: occlusion.

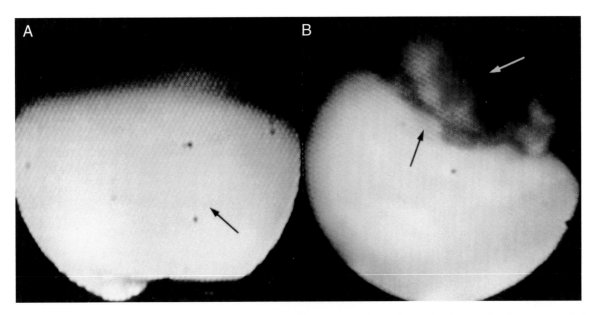

Fig. 3. Angioscopic images of the same patient as in Fig. 2. Glistening yellow plaque in the proximal segment of the RCA before (**A**) and globular red thrombus (white arrow) on the disrupted identical plaque (black arrow) 3 hours after the onset of the attack (**B**).

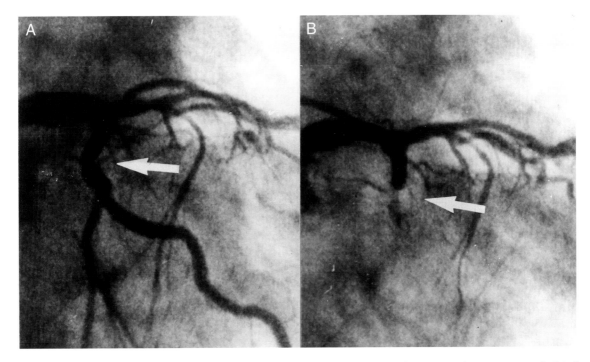

Fig. 4. S.H., 70-year-old male. **A:** before acute myocardial infarction. **B:** 4 hours after onset of acute myocardial infarction.

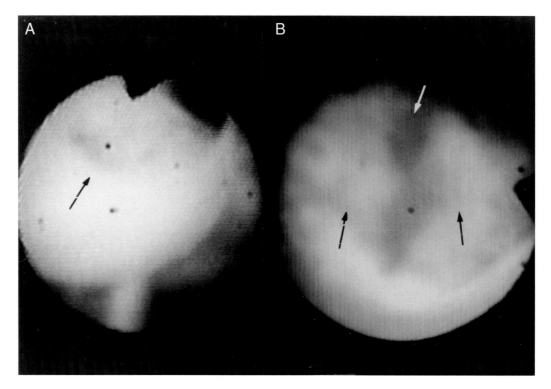

Fig. 5. Angioscopic images of the same patient as in Fig. 4. **A:** erosion on a white plaque before acute myocardial infarction (arrow). **B:** disruption of the identical plaque (black arrows) and thrombus on it (white arrow) 4 hours after onset of acute myocardial infarction.

Reference

1. Uchida Y, Nakamura F, Tomaru T, et al: Prediction of acute coronary syndromes by percutaneous coronary angioscopy in patients with stable angina. Am Heart J 130:195–203, 1995.

Chapter 17

Stabilization of Vulnerable Atherosclerotic Coronary Plaques

If vulnerable coronary plaques are removed or stabilized (regressed) by any means, it is a great benefit to human beings. There are at least 3 possible approaches for plaque stabilization: in addition to endothelial cell stabilization, reduction of lipid deposited in the plaque and collagen fiber growth in the fibrous cap, positive remodeling (increase in vessel diameter) with collagen fiber growth in the cap, and mechanical removal of the plaque (Fig. 1).

Medical Stabilization of Vulnerable Coronary Plaques

Since long-term administration of antihyperlipidemic agents results in reduction of cardiac events and increases survival rate, it is generally believed that antihyperlipidemic agents can stabilize vulnerable coronary plaques.[1-3] However, coronary angiographic follow-up studies demonstrated that their beneficial effects are not necessarily accompanied by a significant reduction in the severity of coronary stenoses.[4-7]

Recent pathological and angioscopic studies revealed that vulnerability of coronary plaques is not related to severity of stenoses and that the rims rather than top of the plaques disrupt.[8,9] Also, angioscopic studies in acute coronary syndromes demonstrated that plaques in less stenotic portions disrupt in a certain group of patients.[10] Therefore, angiography is not adequate for evaluation of vulnerability.

Angioscopy enables macroscopic pathological evaluation of the coronary plaques. Therefore, we carried out a prospective angioscopic open trial for evaluation of the stabilizing effects of an antihyperlipidemic agent with bezafibrate. The plaques were classified as white, light yellow, white and nonglistening yellow on mosaic, nonglistening yellow (rarely brown), and glistening yellow.[11-13] Also, they were classified as regular (nondisrupted) and complex (disrupted) plaques.[13,14] Our angioscopic and pathological studies revealed that glistening yellow plaques are the most vulnerable and yellow ones are the next most vulnerable, as described in detail in Chapter 5.

Therefore, the vulnerability score of plaques was determined based on their color and surface morphology and it was compared before and 6 months later (Table 1). In Fig. 1A, a glistening yellow complex (rough-surfaced) plaque was changed into a nonglistening yellow regular plaque (vulnerability score changed from 4 to 2). In Fig. 1B, a nonglistening yellow regular plaque disappeared almost completely and the luminal surface became white (vulnerability score changed from 2 to 0). In Fig. 1C, a yellow and brown plaque was reduced in size and the neighboring surface changed from light yellow into white (vulnerability score from 2 to 1).

Thus, the vulnerability score was reduced (from 1.6 to 0.8; P<0.05) in the bezafibrate group and was unchanged (from 1.4 to 1.3; NS) in the control group (Fig. 2). Two or more plaques with a vulnerability score of 1 or more were observed in 4 patients who were treated. In 2 of these patients, the vulnerability score was decreased in one plaque but was unchanged in others (Fig. 3), suggesting different susceptibility of plaques to this agent even in the same patient.

Total cholesterol was unchanged, triglycerides were decreased, and high-density lipoproteins were increased in the bezafibrate group but were unchanged in the control group (Fig. 4). The results of this study indicate a possibility that 6 months of oral administration of bezafibrate can reduce the vulnerability score (Fig. 5).[15] Further double-blind studies with various categories of agents such as antihyperlipidemic, anti-inflammatory, and antioxidant agents are required to clarify what kind of agent is the most effective for stabilization of vulnerable coronary plaques.

Possible Ways for Plaque Stabilization

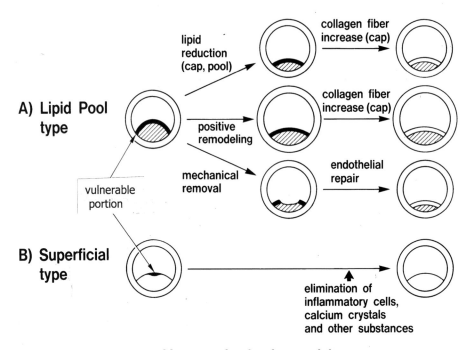

Fig. 1. Possible approaches for plaque stabilization.

Table 1
Angioscopic Vulnerability Score of Coronary Plaques

	score
1) Plaque color	
White	0
Light yellow	1
Yellow and white on mosaic	1
Nonglistening yellow	2
Glistening yellow	3
2) Surface morphology	
Smooth	0
Irregular	1

Removal or Stabilization of Vulnerable Plaques by Interventional Therapy

We started to clarify whether the glistening yellow plaques, which we believe to be most vulnerable, can be stabilized by balloon angioplasty, directional atherectomy, or stents.

Fig. 6 shows a glistening yellow plaque that was found in the left circumflex (LCx) artery. Plain old balloon angioplasty (POBA) was performed on this plaque to artificially disrupt it and, as a consequence, to prevent spontaneous disruption and, accordingly, to prevent spontaneous disruption and, accordingly, acute coronary syndromes. Three months later, however, restenosis occurred. Angioscopy revealed a relatively smooth plaque. The portion where the glistening yellow plaque existed before was now light yellow in color. POBA was performed on this restenotic segment. Again 3 months later, restenosis was not observed and the luminal surface was bluish white and reflected illumination, indicating regenerated endothelial cells covering the surface (Fig. 6). The results suggest that interventional therapy is one choice for elimination of vulnerable plaques and accordingly for prevention of acute coronary syndromes in patients with this category of vulnerable plaques.

One serious unresolved problem is restenosis that frequently occurs following interventions. Another problem is that it is controversial to perform interventions on the plaques in segments with insignificant stenosis. Nevertheless, when characterization of the vulnerable plaque by any means is established, it may be acceptable to remove it by interventions to prevent these fatal syndromes.

Since angioscopy is an interventional and rather subjective diagnostic tool, other noninterventional and more objective tools, including measurement of plasma factors that selectively reflect vulnerability and also noninterventional therapeutic means, should be developed in the future to minimize the great burden acute coronary syndromes place on humans.

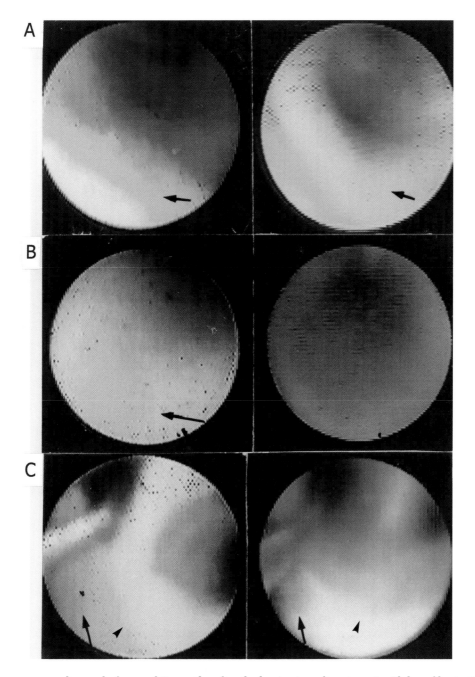

Fig. 2. Changes in coronary plaques before and 6 months after the beginning of treatment with bezafibrate. **Left:** before treatment. **Right:** 6 months after treatment. **A:** T.H., 60-year-old male. A glistening yellow plaque in segment 13 before it was changed into a yellow plaque 6 months later. **B:** M.T., 67-year-old male. A nonglistening yellow plaque in segment 3 before it disappeared (or was absorbed?) 6 months later. **C:** K.M., 61-year-old male. A yellow plaque was reduced in size (arrow) and the surrounding portions changed from light yellow into bluish white (arrowhead).

Changes in Vulnerability Score

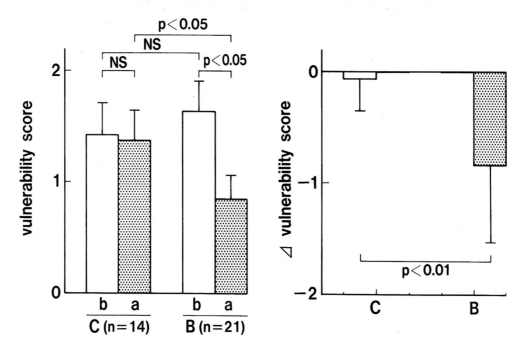

Fig. 3. Changes in vulnerability score. b: before. a: 6 months after. **C:** control group. **B:** bezafibrate group. NS: not significant.

Differential Effects of Bezafibrate on Plaque in the Same Patients

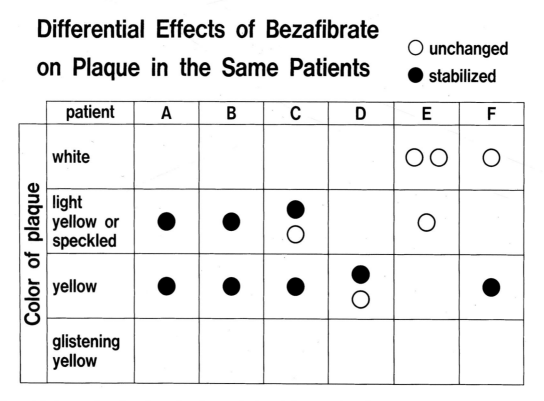

Fig. 4. Differential changes in color of regular plaques (vulnerability score) in the same patients. Open circle: unchanged. Solid black circle: reduced in score.

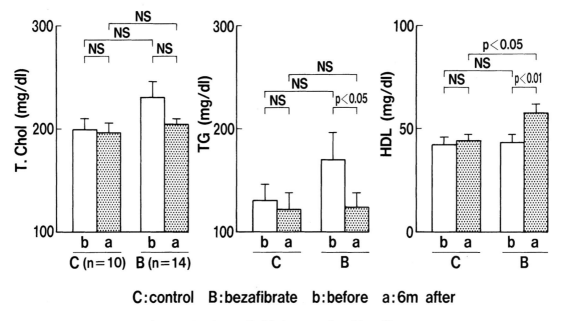

C:control   B:bezafibrate   b:before   a:6m after

Fig. 5. Changes in plasma lipids in control and bezafibrate groups.

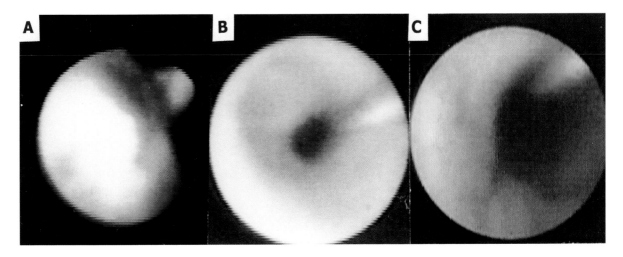

Fig. 6. H.T., 58-year-old male. Angioscopic images of the POBA site. A: a glistening yellow plaque before POBA. B: restenosis after 3 months. The portion where the glistening yellow plaque existed was light yellow. C: 3 months after re-POBA. Bluish white luminal surface.

References

1. Waters D, Higgins L, Gladstone P: Effect of lovastatin upon the evolution of coronary atherosclerosis as assessed by serial quantitative coronary arteriography. J Am Coll Cardiol 21:1312–1318, 1993.
2. The Scandinavian Simvastatin Survival Study Group: Randomised trial of cholesterol lowering in 4444 patients with coronary heart disease: the Scandinavian Simvastatin Survival Study (4S). Lancet 344:138, 1993.
3. Shepherd J, Cobbe SM, Ford I, et al: Prevention of coronary heart disease with pravastatin in men with hypercholesterolemia. N Engl J Med 333:1301–1307, 1995.
4. Jakema JW, Bruschke AVG, van Boven T, REGRESS

Study Group: Effects of lipid lowering by pravastatin on progression and regression of coronary artery disease in symptomatic men with normal to moderately elevated serum cholesterol levels. Circulation 91:2528–2540, 1995.

5. Ericsson CG, Hamsten A, Nilsson J, et al: Angiographic assessment of effects of bezafibrate on progression of coronary artery disease in young male post-infarction patients. Lancet 347:849–853, 1996.

6. Ericsson CG, Nilsson J, Grip L, Svane B, et al: Effects of bezafibrate treatment of five years on coronary plaques causing 20% to 50% diameter narrowings (The Bezafibrate Atherosclerosis Intervention Trial). Am J Cardiol 80:1125–1129, 1997.

7. Ericsson CG: Results of the bezafibrate coronary atherosclerosis trial (BECAIT) and an update on trials now in progress. Eur Heart J 19:H37–41, 1998.

8. Yutani C, Hao H: Histopathological study of acute myocardial infarction and pathology of coronary thrombosis: A comparative study in four districts in Japan. Jpn Circ J 51:352, 1987.

9. Hao H, Yutani N: Histopathological aspects of coronary thrombosis and its progression. In: Coronary Clinics. 1994, pp 121–127.

10. Uchida Y, Nakamura F, Tomaru T, et al: Prediction of acute coronary syndromes by percutaneous coronary angioscopy in patients with stable angina. Am Heart J 130:204–211, 1995.

11. Uchida Y, Kanai M, Uchida H, et al: Angioscopic classification of coronary plaques and its pathological correlations. Coronary 16:302–313, 1999.

12. Uchida Y, Takeuchi K, Kanai M, et al: Glistening yellow plaque, a vulnerable plaque, and its pathological correlations. Circulation 100(Suppl 1):514, 1999.

13. Uchida Y: Angioscopic detection of vulnerable plaques and prediction of acute coronary syndromes. In: The Vulnerable Atherosclerotic Plaque, Futura Publishing Co., Armonk, NY, 1999.

14. Sherman CT, Litback F, Grundfest W: Coronary angioscopy in patients with unstable angina pectoris. New Engl J Med 315:913–919, 1986.

15. Uchida Y, Fujimori Y, Ohsawa H, et al: Angioscopic evaluation of stabilizing effects of bezafibrate on coronary plaques. Coronary 16:293–301, 1999.

PART II

Clinical Application of Percutaneous Cardioscopy for Coronary Heart Disease

Chapter 18

History of
Percutaneous Cardioscopy:

An Overview of the Literature

Coronary microvessel disease is another important category of ischemic heart disease. However, direct visualization of the microvessels is beyond conventional angioscopy. Assessment of the changes in regional myocardial blood flow secondary to the epicardial coronary artery disease is also important in the diagnosis and treatment of ischemic heart disease. Although used clinically, contrast echocardiography, radioisotope imaging, positron emission tomography, and contrast angiography are indirect modalities of diagnosis and they are not feasible for instantaneous assessment of microcirculation of the heart.

There are at least 3 possible approaches for direct observation of the coronary microvessels and regional myocardial blood flow: through the endocardial surface, through the epicardial surface, and within the myocardium.

Intracardiac observation by a rigid cardioscope in animals was reported by Allen in 1922 and by Harken in 1943. In 1956, Sakakibara and his coworkers used a rigid cardioscope for observation of an atrial septal defect during open heart surgery (Fig. 1). They also observed aortic valves using the same cardioscope in 1958. The images they obtained were very beautiful.

Due to difficulty in manufacturing a thin endoscope that can be safely introduced percutaneously into the cardiac chambers and equipment for displacement of blood, approximately 29 years elapsed until Uchida and his coworkers successfully performed percutaneous cardioscopy in patients. Although this new modality of diagnosis is now performed routinely in selected institutions, it is still not used worldwide.

Previously reported papers on percutaneous cardioscopy are listed below.

Animal Experiments

Allen DS, Graham EA: Intracardiac surgery: A new method. Am Med Assoc 79:1028, 1922.

Harken DE, Glidden EM: Experiments in intracardiac surgery. II. Intracardiac visualization. J Thorac Surg 12:566, 1943.

Uchida Y, Tomaru T, Nakamura F, Sonoki H, Sugimoto T: Fiberoptic angioscopy of cardiac chambers, valves and great vessels using a guiding balloon catheter in dog. Am Heart J 118:1297–1302,1988.

Uchida Y, Nakamura F, Tsukamoto T, You S, Kido H, Sugimoto T: Percutaneous ventricular endomyocardial biopsy with angioscopic guidance. Am Heart J 118:1039–1041,1989.

Nakamura F, Uchida Y, Tomaru T, Kamijo T, Sugimoto T: Laser ablation of myocardium with angioscopic guidance. Circulation (Suppl)1990 (abstract).

Uchida Y: Cardioscope-guided intracardiac surgery. Op Nursing 6:16–22, 1991 (in Japanese).

Uchida Y, Nakamura F, Kido H, Sugimoto T: Percutaneous cardiomyotomy and valvulotomy with angioscopic guidance. Am Heart J 121:1221–1224, 1991.

Uchida Y, Tomaru T, Nakamura F, Miwa A, Kamijo T: Transcatheter treatment of hypertrophic obstructive cardiomyopathy. Jpn Circulat J (Suppl):130, 1991 (in Japanese).

Clinical Applications

During Open Heart Surgery

Sakakibara H, Ichikawa T, Hattori J: An intraoperative method for observation of cardiac septal de-

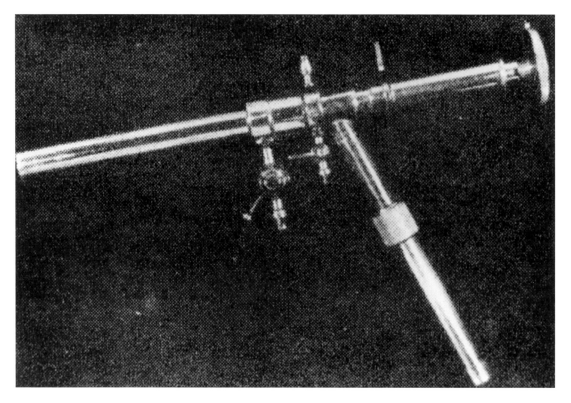

Fig. 1. A rigid endoscope used by Sakakibara for observation of the cardiac chambers during open heart surgery.

fect using a cardioscope. Operation 10:285–290, 1956 (in Japanese).

Sakaibara H, Iijima T, Hattori J, Inomata K: Direct visual operation for aortic stenosis: Cardioscope studies. J Int Coll Surg 29:548, 1958.

Percutaneous

Uchida Y, Ohshima T, Shibuya I: Percutaneous angioscopy of the right side of the heart in humans. Cardiovasc World Report 1:13–17,1988.

Uchida Y, Oshima T, Fujimori Y: Observation of the left ventricle in patients with dilated cardiomyopathy and acute myocarditis. Proceedings of Japanese College of Cardiology, 1989.

Uchida Y: Percutaneous cardiovascular angioscopy. In: Lasers in Cardiovascular Medicine and Surgery. Abela G (ed). Kluwer Academic Press, Boston, 1989, pp 399–410.

Uchida Y, Fujimori Y, Hirose J: Percutaneous left ventricular endomyocardial biopsy with angioscopic guidance in patients with dilated cardiomyopathy. Am Heart J 119:949–952,1990.

Uchida Y, Nakamura F, Ohshima T, Fujimori Y, Hirose J: Percutaneous fiberoptic angioscopy of the left ventricle in patients with dilated cardiomyopathy and acute myocarditis. Am Heart J 120:677–687, 1990.

Uchida Y, Ohshima T, Yoshihara F, Fujimori Y, Hirose J, Mukai H, Kawashima M: Percutaneous fiberoptic angioscopy of cardiac valves. Am Heart J 121:1791–1798, 1991.

Uchida Y: Percutaneous angioscopy of cardiac chambers and valves. In: Progress in Cardiology. Zipes D (ed). Lea & Febiger, Boston, 1991, pp 163–192.

Hirose J, Fujimori Y, Ooshima T, Uchida Y: Observation of the left ventricle in patients with rheumatic heart disease. Cardioangioscopy and Laser Cardioangioplasty, 30, 1991 (in Japanese).

Fujimori Y, Oshima T, Hirose J, Uchida Y: Cardioscopic features of left ventricle in patients with idiopathic hypertrophic cardiomyopathy. Cardioangioscopy and Laser Cardioangioplasty, 28, 1991 (in Japanese).

Uchida Y, Fujimori Y, Hirose J: Percutaneous cardioscopy. Jpn Heart J 33:271–294, 1992.

Uchida Y: Effects of nitroglycerin and nicorandil on subendocardial blood flow in patients with ischemic heart disease. Therapeutic Res 13:93–99, 1992 (in Japanese).

Hirose J, Sasaki S, Morizuki M, Ohshima T, Takahashi M, Tsubouchi H, Uchida Y: Follow-up study of patients with idiopathic myocarditis by percutaneous cardioscopy. Cardioangioscopy and Laser Cardioangioplasty 4:33–34, 1995 (in Japanese).

Oshima T, Hirose J, Sasaki M, Morizuki M, Takahashi M, Uchida Y: Detection of mural thrombus of cardiac chambers by percutaneous cardioscopy. Cardioangioscopy and Laser Cardioangioplasty 4:35–36, 1995 (in Japanese).

Uchida Y: Atlas of Cardioangioscopy. Medical View, Tokyo, 1995.

Uchida Y, Kanai M, Ohsawa H, Uchi T, Noike H: Direct visualization of subendocardial microvessels by percutaneous cardioscopy in patients with heart disease. Circulation 98(Suppl):I-448,1998 (abstract).

Uchida Y, Kanai M, Sakura T: Discrimination of left ventricular myocardial layers by an intracardiac ultrasonography in patients with ischemic heart disease. Jpn Circ J 64(Suppl I):172, 2000.

Chapter 19

Developmental History of Cardioscopes

In 1975, a 9 F fiberscope was developed in collaboration with Olympus Co., Tokyo. The fiberscope was introduced through an 11 F hard-tipped guiding catheter into the canine left ventricle (Fig. 1A). This cardioscope was abandoned due to marked damage onto the endocardial surface. In 1976, a 10 F balloon-tipped guiding catheter was developed. This catheter allowed a 6 F fiberscope to pass through. However, this cardioscope was abandoned because the balloon became frosty during observation due to temperature difference between the saline used for balloon dilatation and the blood in the ventricle (Fig. 1B). In the same year, a fiberscope with a balloon fixed on the distal-most tip was devised. This fiberscope had a central lumen through which warmed body-temperature saline could be infused for dilatation of the balloon. The balloon was pushed against the endocardial surface to observe the changes through the dilated balloon (Figs. 1B and 2A). However, introduction of this fiberscope alone into the left ventricle is very difficult because a guidewire cannot be used, and when used in combination with a guiding catheter, a big guiding catheter must be used to allow the fiberscope to pass through. Therefore, this fiberscope is not used clinically. Shure used this type of fiberscope for observation of the pulmonary artery in patients.[1]

In 1983, a 9 F guiding balloon catheter was devised in collaboration with Clinical Supply Co., Gifu, Japan. When inflated with CO_2, the balloon protruded more distally than the shaft tip to form a dead space between the target and the balloon and also to prevent myocardial damages by the shaft tip. In combination with a 5 F fiberscope, this balloon catheter enabled percutaneous transluminal observation of the cardiac chambers and valves (Figs. 1D and 2B).[2] This cardioscopy system is now routinely used clinically for observation not only of the cardiac chambers and valves[2] but also of the pulmonary artery[3] and aorta.[4] In this guiding balloon catheter, preshaping of the tip is required for observation of the desired portions of the heart. Therefore, a guiding catheter with a soft tip and a tip-bending devise was developed in 1993. This cardioscopy system enabled observation of the desired portions in the heart.[4]

In 1994, a 7 F cardioscope for single use was devised. This angioscope had a balloon at the distal-most tip and had 3 channels, in one of which a fiberscope was fixed so as to locate its distal tip to the catheter tip. The other 2 channels were used for guidewire insertion and for saline flush, respectively. Although this cardioscope does not require a guiding catheter, preshaping of the tip is difficult. Therefore, this cardioscope is infrequently used.

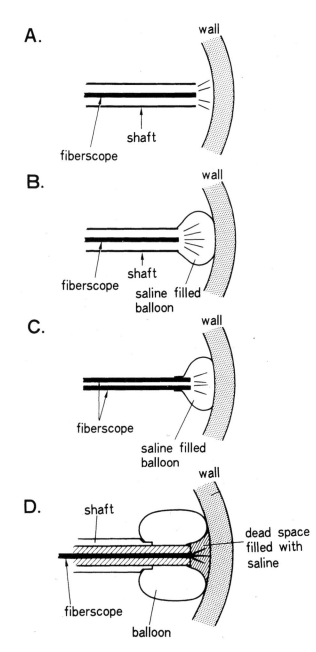

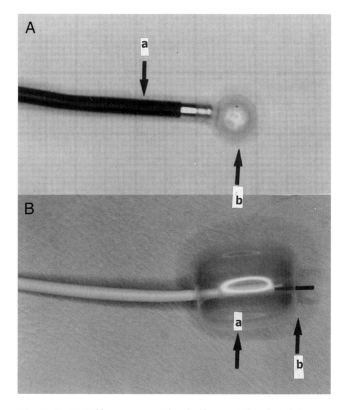

Fig. 1. Schematic representation of the cardioscopes previously developed in our laboratories.

Fig. 2. A: 10 F fiberscope with a balloon at the distal tip. **a:** shaft. **b:** balloon. **B:** 9 F guiding balloon catheter with a steerable fiberscope inside. **a:** balloon. **b:** fiberscope.

References

1. Shure S, Gregoratos G, Mose MM: Angioscopy is useful in evaluation of chronic pulmonary arterial obstruction. Circulation 70(Suppl II):182, 1984.
2. Uchida Y: Percutaneous cardiovascular angioscopy. In: Lasers in Cardiovascular Medicine and Surgery. Abela G (ed). Kluwer Academic Publishers, Boston, 1989, pp 399–410.
3. Uchida Y, Ohshima T, Shibuya I: Percutaneous angioscopy of the right side of the heart in humans. Cardiovasc World Report 1:13–17, 1988.
4. Uchida Y: Atlas of Cardioangioscopy. Medical View, Tokyo, 1995.

Chapter 20

Percutaneous Cardioscopy Systems and Their Manipulation

Fiberoptic examinations, as recently demonstrated in coronary, pulmonary,[1] and peripheral vessels,[2] allow direct observation of pathology not otherwise obtainable. Recently, similar techniques have been applied to examine all of the cardiac chambers and valves in patients with various categories of heart disease.[3-5]

Cardioscopy System

The cardioscopy system is essentially the same as that used for coronary angioscopy. It is composed of a cardioscope (fiberscope and guiding catheter), CCD camera and its amplifier, illumination source, image mixer, video recorder (either tape or DVD), and monitor. Both cardioscopic and x-ray images are displayed simultaneously on a monitor and are recorded through the mixer on the recorder for identification of the observed target (see Chapter 3).

Clinically Used Cardioscopes

The cardioscope is composed of a 4.2 F fiberscope with 4000 image fibers and 200 illumination fibers (Olympus Co., Tokyo, Japan) and either a 9 F guiding balloon catheter with or without a tip-bending device (Clinical Supply Co., Gifu, Japan) or a 8 F or 9 F soft-tipped guiding catheter with a tip-bending device without a balloon (Olympus Co.) (Fig. 1).

In the case of a guiding balloon catheter without a tip-bending device, the tip configuration is preshaped, depending on the location of the target for observation. Configuration of the guiding balloon catheter tip and the observable target sites are shown in Fig. 2. Two to 3.5 mL of carbon dioxide is required to fully inflate the balloon. The diameter of the visual field obtained is 5–10 mm in water. In the case of a soft-tipped guiding

catheter with a bending device, the manipulator at the proximal end, which is connected to the metallic ring at the distal-most tip with a stainless steel wire, is pulled to bend the catheter tip (Fig. 1C).

Cardioscope-Guided Endomyocardial Biopsy Catheter

To correlate the cardioscopic images to the histological changes in the observed target, we developed a cardioscope-guided endomyocardial biopsy.[5] A 1.6 F fiberscope and a bioptome are introduced through either the 9 F guiding balloon catheter or a 9 F soft-tipped catheter into the heart (Figs. 3, 4). Biopsy is performed during saline infusion for confirmation of the target to be biopsied (Fig. 5).

Sterilization

Before use, the fiberscope is sterilized with ethylene oxide gas (EOG). Guiding catheters are also sterilized with EOG and are packed for immediate use.

Premedication

Premedication is the same as that for coronary angioscopy (see Chapter 3).

Procedures

Observation of the Left Ventricle Using a Guiding Balloon Catheter

After routine left ventriculography at RAO and LAO projections for determination of the wall seg-

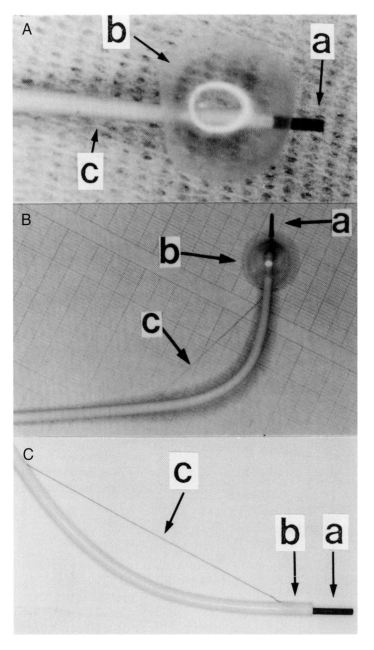

Fig. 1. Cardioscopes devised in our laboratories **A:** 9 F guiding balloon catheter and 5 F fiberscope. **a:** fiberscope. **b:** balloon. **c:** shaft. **B:** 9 F guiding balloon catheter with bending device. **a:** fiberscope. **b:** balloon. **c:** stainless steel wire for bending. **C:** 9 F guiding catheter with bending device. **a:** fiberscope. **b:** shaft. C: stainless steel wire for tip bending.

ments to be observed, 50 mg xylocaine is injected intravenously for arrhythmia prophylaxis. Then, a 9 F guiding balloon catheter is advanced through the 9 F sheath previously introduced through the right femoral artery into the left ventricle guided by a guidewire. Use of a 0.035 Radiofocus guidewire with J configuration (Termo Co., Tokyo, Japan) is recommended for smooth introduction of the guiding catheter. Immediately after introduction of the catheter into the desired segment of the left ventricle,

the balloon is inflated with carbon dioxide to prevent tissue damage by the catheter shaft tip, and then the guidewire is removed. Balloon size is changed by controlling the amount of carbon dioxide, depending on the curvature and trabeculae of the wall segment to be observed. Then, a fiberscope is advanced through the guiding catheter so as to locate its tip a few millimeters proximal to the catheter tip to prevent tissue damage caused by friction between the fiberscope tip and the ventricular wall. The guiding

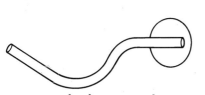

**apical segment,
inferior segment,
anterior segment**

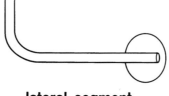

lateral segment

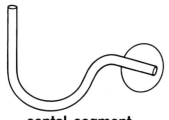

**septal segment,
anterior segment**

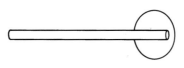

**high posterior
segment**

Fig. 2. Schematic representation of the tip configuration of the guiding balloon catheter and left ventricular segments to be observed.

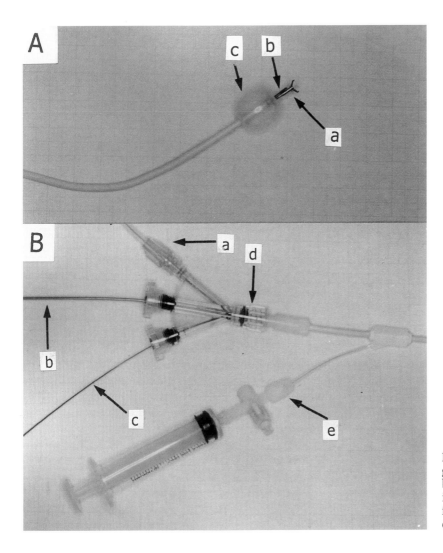

Fig. 3. Cardioscope-guided bioptome with guiding balloon catheter. **A:** catheter tip. **a:** bioptome. **b:** fiberscope. **c:** balloon. **B:** proximal end. **a:** flush channel. **b:** bioptome. **c:** fiberscope. **d:** duostat. **e:** balloon inflation channel.

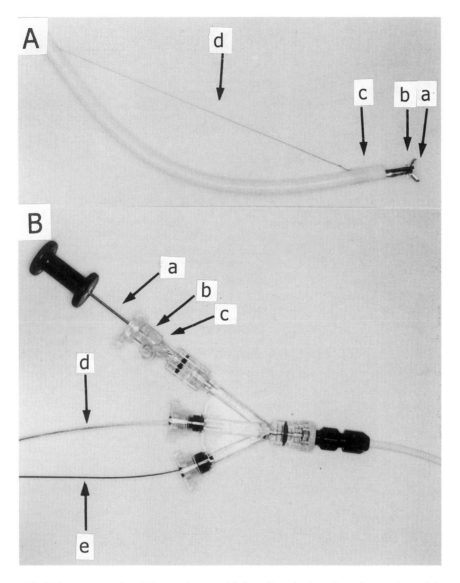

Fig. 4. Cardioscope-guided bioptome and guiding catheter with bending device. **A:** catheter tip. **a:** bioptome. **b:** fiberscope. **c:** shaft. **d:** stainless steel wire. **B:** proximal end of catheter. **a:** bending controller. **b:** stopper. **c:** flush channel. **d:** bioptome. **e:** fiberscope.

balloon catheter is manipulated under fluoroscopy so that the balloon is directly contiguous with the portion targeted for examination.

The balloon is pushed against the endocardial surface to make a dead space between the balloon and the endocardium. Upon pushing the balloon so it touches the endocardium, ventricular arrhythmias always occur. However, they disappear spontaneously within a few seconds. When the balloon touches and then detaches from the endocardial surface, arrhythmias do not disappear. In this case, balloon size should be reduced so it continues to touch the endocardial surface.

Then, heparinized (heparin 10 IU/mL) saline

warmed to body temperature is infused by a power injector at a rate of 5 mL/sec for displacement of the blood in the dead space for observation. When observation of more than one segment is necessary, we observe the anterior first, using a preshaped guiding balloon catheter. After observation of the anterior wall, the catheter is pulled back and the apical segment is observed. Then the catheter is rotated counterclockwise to observe the lateral wall. The catheter is then pulled back further and rotated clockwise or counterclockwise to observe the inferior and posterior wall segments (Fig. 6).

When blood displacement is incomplete, partial reduction in balloon size should be considered. After

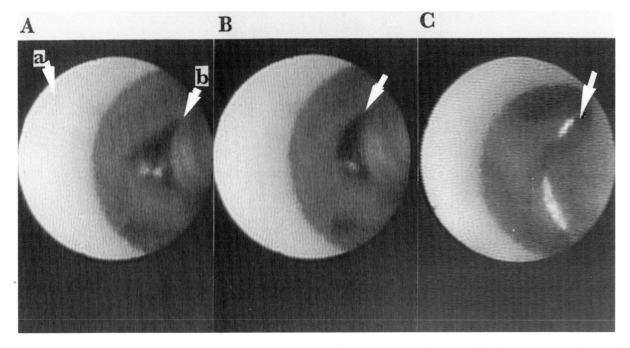

Fig. 5. Process of cardioscope-guided endomyocardial biopsy. **A:** during opening of cusps of the bioptome. **a:** catheter shaft. **b:** bioptome. **B:** during closure of the cusps.

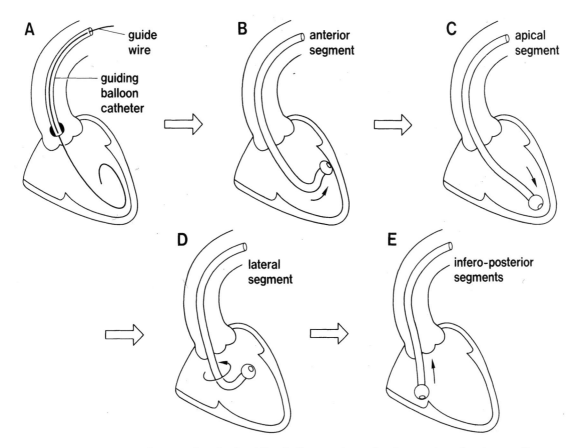

Fig. 6. Schematic representation of manipulation of guiding balloon catheter for observation of various wall segments of the left ventricle.

observation is complete, the fiberscope is replaced by a thinner fiberscope and a bioptome, shown in Fig. 3, for cardioscope-guided endomyocardial biopsy. After each observation or biopsy, contrast material is injected in order to document the portions under inspection.

After biopsy is complete, the balloon is pulled back down to the descending aorta without balloon deflation. Although not experienced in our laboratories, deflation of the balloon in the left ventricle or the ascending aorta may cause detachment of the thrombus that might be formed on the balloon, resulting in cerebral or coronary thromboembolism.

Observation of the Left Ventricle Using a Guiding Catheter With a Bending Device

A soft-tipped 8 F or 9 F guiding balloon catheter with a bending device is also used for cardioscopy and endomyocardial biopsy. The catheter is introduced, guided by a 0.035 Radiofocus guidewire, into the left ventricle. The guidewire is replaced by a fiberscope. Then, the catheter tip is bent by controlling the manipulator appropriate for observation of the desired portion (Fig. 7). Endomyocardial biopsy is also performed using the device shown in Fig. 5.

After the observation or biopsy is complete, the guiding catheter is reshaped in straight configuration by controlling the bending device and pulled back.

Observation of the Right Heart

A 9 F guiding balloon catheter in a U configuration is introduced through the femoral vein into the right ventricle, and then a 5 F fiberscope is introduced through the catheter into the right ventricle. The balloon is inflated and pushed against the outflow tract, septum, apical, and then posterobasal wall segments for observation. After each observation, contrast material is injected to confirm the observed portion. Thereafter, the fiberscope and guiding balloon catheter are pulled back to the right atrium, and the atrial wall and septum are similarly observed.[6]

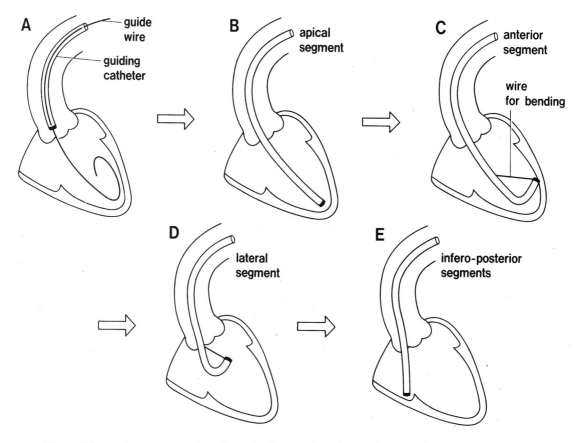

Fig. 7. Schematic representation of manipulation of guiding catheter with tip-bending device.

Dye Image Cardioscopy for Identification of Endocardial Damage and Evaluation of Myocardial Blood Flow

Dye image cardioscopy can be performed for identification of endothelial damages, estimation of myocardial blood flow, and for other purposes.[7] Evans blue, which is used for the coronary artery, is used for discrimination of endocardial damage in various categories of heart disease, because in addition to flow stagnation, existence of endocardial damage accelerates thrombus formation in the cardiac chambers. After routine observation of a given wall segment, 1 mL of 2% Evans blue solution is injected through the guiding catheter into the ventricle. Then, saline is again infused to observe whether the segment is stained in blue or not. Special care is required so that the balloon does not dislocate; otherwise, the endocardium of the observed segment is damaged and stained, leading to misinterpretation.

When the same dose of Evans blue is injected into the coronary artery, the segment irrigated by the artery and therefore patency of the irrigating artery can be examined. Special attention should be directed to the patient's condition, because this dye occasionally causes anaphylaxis.

Fluorescent Image Cardioscopy

The illumination source is equipped with various fluorescence excitation filters. Also, exchangeable cut filters are incorporated in the ICCD for fluorescent images.

Cardioscopy after selective intracoronary injection of 1 mL of 1% fluorescein isothiocyanate conjugated (FITC) reveals whether or not blood is supplied or not to the observed segment.

Adjustment of Illumination

The cardioscopy system manufactured by Olympus Co. is equipped with a controller for graded illumination output. Therefore, semiquantitative control of illumination output can be obtained.

Calibration

When calibration of the target is required, a 0.014-inch guidewire is introduced simultaneously with the fiberscope into the cardiac chamber for calibration of the target (Fig. 8).

Complications

Guiding Balloon Catheter

Major complications that may occur are rupture of the balloon and consequent coronary and cerebral gas embolism, and coronary and cerebral thromboembolism with the thrombus formed on the balloon catheter in the endocardium. In our consecutive 200 patients who underwent left ventricular cardioscopy, an abrupt elevation of the ST segment on the electrocardiogram occurred in 2 patients. Immediate coronary angiography revealed occlusion of the LAD with gas leaked from the balloon in one and coronary spasm in the other patient. Cerebral accident was observed in no patients. Endocardial bleeding was frequently observed as a minor complication, probably due to friction between the protruded fiberscope tip and the endocardial surface (Fig. 9).

Ventricular arrhythmias occurred in all patients upon pushing the balloon against the wall. However, the arrhythmias subsided within a few seconds.

Guiding Catheter With a Bending Device

No serious complications were noted except mechanically induced endocardial bleeding. In one patient, kinking of the soft portion of the catheter shaft occurred and advancement of the fiberscope was disturbed. Introduction of a 0.014-inch guidewire with the fiberscope prevented kinking.

What Should and Should Not Be Done

1. Before use, gas leakage should be examined by inflating the balloon of the guiding catheter in saline.
2. The fiberscope tip should not be advanced outside the guiding catheter shaft during observation. Although the tip is smooth and flexible, the fiber-

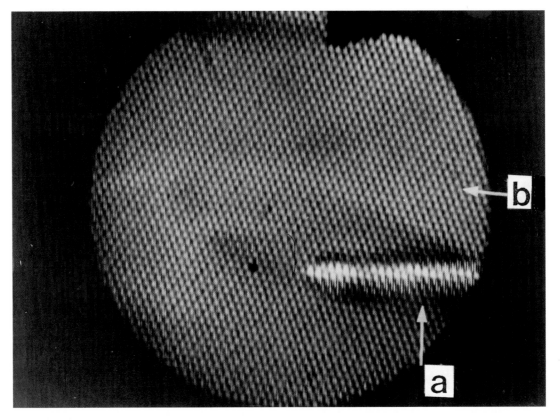

Fig. 8. Calibration of the size of the target using a 0.014-inch guidewire as a reference. **a:** trabeculae. **b:** guidewire.

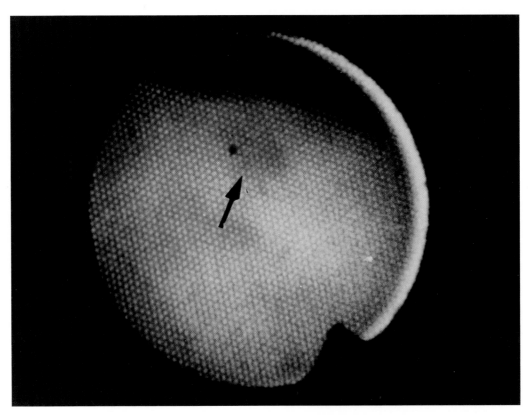

Fig. 9. Endocardial bleeding induced by the fiberscope tip (arrow).

scope may damage the ventricular wall by friction or penetration. When the fiberscope tip touches the endocardial surface, halation occurs. On such occasions, the fiberscope should be pulled back a few millimeters.

3. Replace the guiding balloon catheter when the balloon shrinks during inflation because it means gas leakage.

4. After observation is complete, pull the guiding balloon catheter back down to the descending aorta without deflating the balloon. Otherwise, the thrombus formed on the balloon might be detached and cause coronary or cerebral embolism.

5. The guiding catheter with the bending device should not be pulled back at the bent configuration; otherwise, damage to the chordae, papillary muscles, and valves by the stainless steel wire may occur.

References

1. Uchida Y, Oshima T, Hirose J, et al: Angioscopic detection of residual pulmonary thrombi in the differential diagnosis of pulmonary embolism. Am Heart J 130:854–859, 1995.
2. Uchida Y, Fujimori Y, Tomaru T, et al: Percutaneous angioplasty of chronic obstruction of peripheral arteries by a temperature controlled Nd:YAG laser system. J Intervent Cardiol 5:301–308, 1993.
3. Uchida Y: Percutaneous angioscopy of cardiac chambers and valves. In: Progress in Cardiology. Zipes D (ed). Lea & Febiger, Philadelphia, 1991, pp 163–213.
4. Uchida Y, Nakamura F, Oshima T, et al: Percutaneous fiberoptic angioscopy in patients with dilated cardiomyopathy and acute myocarditis. Am Heart J 120:677–687, 1990.
5. Uchida Y, Fujimori Y, Oshima T: Percutaneous cardioscopy. Jpn Heart J 33:271–294, 1992.
6. Uchida Y, Oshima T, Shibuya I: Percutaneous angioscopy of the right side of the heart in humans. Cardiovasc World Rep 1:13–17, 1988.
7. Kanai M, Sakurai T, Uchida Y: Percutaneous dye image cardioscopy for detection of endocardial lesions. Diagn Thera Endoscopy 7:29–34, 2000.

Chapter 21

Intracardiac Ultrasound (ICUS) Probes and Their Manipulation

Percutaneous cardioscopy, as in the case of coronary angioscopy, can evaluate only the surface morphology of the cardiac chambers and valves. Therefore, use of high-resolution ultrasound is necessary for evaluation of the cardiac wall architecture.

Intracardiac Ultrasound (ICUS) Probes

Fig. 1 shows an ICUS probe that we developed in collaboration with Olympus Co. and has been routinely used clinically since 1992. The probe (12, 15, or 20 MHz, 30 rps) is 8 F or 9 F in external diameter, 2 mm long, and has a metallic slider at the distal-most tip for a guidewire to pass through. The metallic slider is angulated at 10° and enables easily passing the probe through an angulated portion such as the aortic arch.

Procedures

Left Ventricle

After observation of the cardiac chamber by cardioscopy, an ICUS probe is introduced through the right femoral artery into the left ventricle, guided by a 0.035-inch guidewire. The guidewire is advanced into the apex first and then the probe is advanced into the apex. Use of a Radiofocus guidewire (Terumo Co., Tokyo) is recommended because it is very steerable. By pulling back the probe slowly, pineapple-like slices of the left ventricle from the apex to the aortic valve can be successively obtained (Fig. 2). ICUS is usually performed after cardioscopy since the ICUS probe may damage the endocardium and may modify cardioscopic images.

A 15-MHz probe is usually used for a normal-sized left ventricle. When the ventricle is large, a 12-MHz probe is used to cover the entire chamber.

Right Ventricle

An ICUS probe is introduced through the right femoral vein into the pulmonary artery guided by a 0.035-inch guidewire. Then, the probe is slowly pulled back toward the right atrium. By this maneuver, pineapple-like slices of the right ventricle can successively be obtained.[1]

Sterilization

Before use, the probe is sterilized with ethylene oxide gas (EOG) as in the case of a cardioscope.

Complications

No complications were noted in 200 successive patients who underwent ICUS in the past. However, vigorous advancement of the probe without a guidewire may cause perforation.

What Should and Should Not Be Done

1. Since the probe is driven mechanically, the probe shaft should not be held vigorously during observation, otherwise the shaft may be broken.
2. During introduction of the probe into the left ventricle, the guidewire tip to the apex should be advanced and then bent to advance along the anterior wall at first, and then the ICUS probe should be advanced, otherwise the probe tip may not be advanced into the apex.

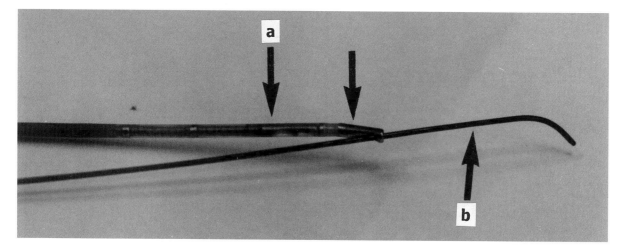

Fig. 1. A 9 F ICUS probe. **a:** shaft. **b:** guidewire. arrow: metallic slider.

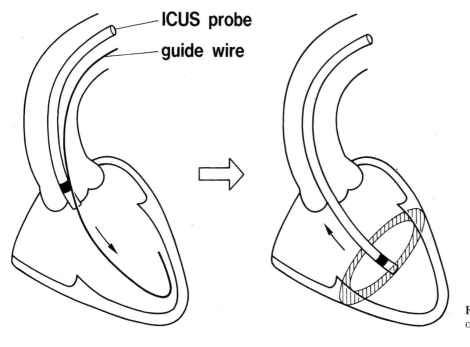

Fig. 2. Schematic representation to observe the left ventricle.

Reference

1. Uchida Y: Atlas of Cardioangioscopy. Medical View Co., Tokyo, 1997.

Chapter 22

Cardiac Chambers in Patients With Ischemic Heart Disease

Normal Heart

Normal Left Ventricle

Anatomically, the left ventricular wall except for the ventricular septum is composed of 3 myocardial layers: the inner oblique, the middle circular, and the outer oblique layers. The inner layer is composed of the free wall and trabeculae. Physiologically, the inner and middle layers contribute mainly to systolic function of the left ventricle while the outer layer connects the right and left ventricles and contributes to systolic ventricular function.

Cardioscopically, the apical wall segment of the normal left ventricle is trabeculated most dominantly, forming trabecular networks. The surface color of the free wall and trabeculae is brown or reddish brown when observed during infusion of saline. The trabeculae become thick and protrude inward during systole (Figs. 1D and 1E). Although less prominent, similar systolic changes are observed in the lateral and inferior wall segments. In the posterior wall segment, the trabeculae are not obvious during diastole. They protrude slightly during systole (Figs. 1F and 1G). The ventricular septum is relatively smooth and light brown in color.[1-3]

The papillary muscles and chordae that connect mitral leaflets to papillary muscles can be easily observed by cardioscopy. The papillary muscles also thicken during systole. The normal chordae are somewhat transparent or German silver-like, reflecting illumination. They are stretched during systole and are relaxed during diastole.[1,2] In contrast to point-to-point observation by cardioscopy, intracardiac ultrasound (ICUS) enables observation of the entire left ventricle within a few minutes. By pulling the ICUS probe back from the ventricular apex toward the aortic valve, pineapple-like slices of the ventricle can be successively obtained (Fig. 2).

In the normal left ventricle, the above-mentioned 3 myocardial layers and the pericardium can be clearly discriminated by ICUS. The 3 layers thicken during each systole. The individual trabeculae that compose the inner layer become thick and fuse with each other during systole and they greatly contribute to reduction of chamber size and, accordingly, to ejection fraction (Fig. 3).[1,4]

Also, aortic cusps are clearly observed by ICUS. The aortic cusp edges are sharp and coapted completely during diastole. They open briskly at early systole, forming at first a triangle-shaped and then a round aortic orifice.[1]

Cardioscopically, the normal aortic cusps are sharp-edged and their surface is smooth and white. They coapt completely during diastole and open briskly at early systole.[3,5]

Lateral projection of both anterior and posterior mitral leaflets can be observed from inside the left ventricle. In particular, the detailed images of the connections between the leaflets and chordae, which are otherwise not obtainable, can be obtained by ICUS.[1]

Cardioscopic observation of the mitral leaflets can be performed either from the left ventricle or from the left atrium.[1] The surface of the normal mitral leaflets are white and smooth. Although irregularly edged, they coapt completely during systole, open briskly at early diastole, and close at early systole forming a dome. At the end of closure, a small amount of the blood is always regurgitated into the left atrium. This may be the cause of mild regurgitation detected by color Doppler ultrasound in the normal heart.

Normal Right Ventricle

Fig. 4 shows venticulographic and cardioscopic images of the normal right ventricle. The luminal surface of the right ventricle is usually brown or reddish

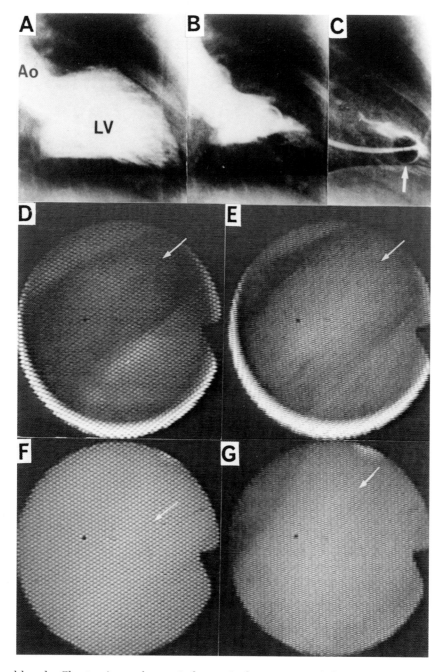

Fig. 1. Y.T., 54-year-old male. Chest pain syndrome. Left ventriculograms at end-diastole (**A**) and end-systole (**B**) and during cardioscopy (**C**). Cardioscopic appearance of the apical segment at end-diastole (**D**) and end-systole (**E**) and inferior segment at end-diastole (**F**) and end-systole (**G**). Arrow in C: guiding balloon catheter. Arrows in D to G: trabeculae. Ao: aorta. LV: left ventricle.

brown but sometimes it is bluish brown due to venous blood. Although less prominent than those of the left ventricle, the trabeculae become thick and protrude inwardly during systole.[6]

By pulling back the ICUS probe from the pulmonary artery toward the right atrium, slices of the outflow and body of right ventricle, atrial septum, membranous and muscular ventricular septa, roots of

the septal leaflet of tricuspid valve and anterior leaflet of mitral valve, papillary muscles, chordae, and finally all 3 tricuspid leaflets can successively be obtained (Fig. 5). Tricuspid leaflets can also be observed by ICUS. The surface of tricuspid leaflets is smooth and white and their edges are sharp. They open briskly at early diastole and close at early systole. As in the case of mitral leaflets, a small amount

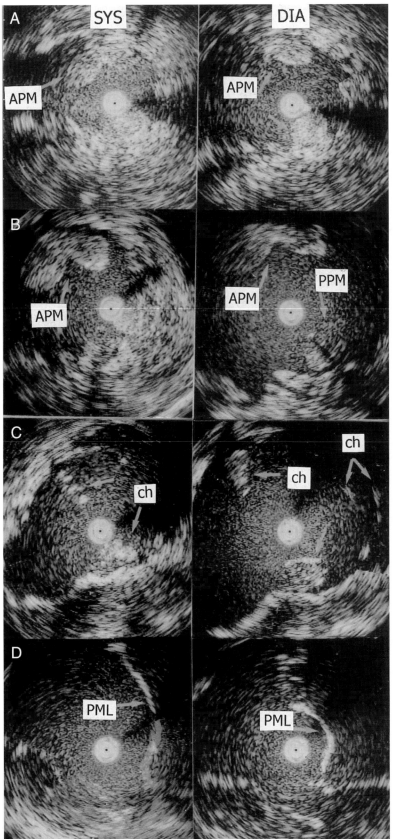

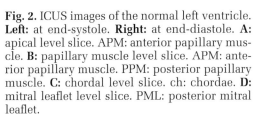

Fig. 2. ICUS images of the normal left ventricle. **Left:** at end-systole. **Right:** at end-diastole. **A:** apical level slice. APM: anterior papillary muscle. **B:** papillary muscle level slice. APM: anterior papillary muscle. PPM: posterior papillary muscle. **C:** chordal level slice. ch: chordae. **D:** mitral leaflet level slice. PML: posterior mitral leaflet.

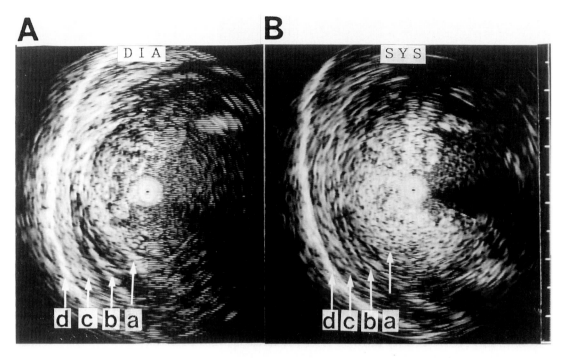

Fig. 3. ICUS images demonstrating normal myocardial layers of the inferior segment of the left ventricle at end-diastole (**A**) and end-systole (**B**). a: inner oblique layer. b: middle circular layer. c: outer oblique layer. d: pericardium.

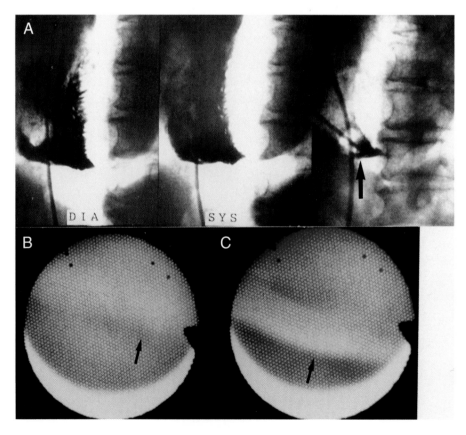

Fig. 4. A, B, and **C:** Right ventriculograms at left anterior oblique projection at end-diastole, end-systole, and during cardioscopic observation of the apical segment, respectively. Arrow in C: guiding balloon catheter. **D** and **E:** cardioscopic images of the apical segment during diastole and systole, respectively. Arrow: trabeculae.

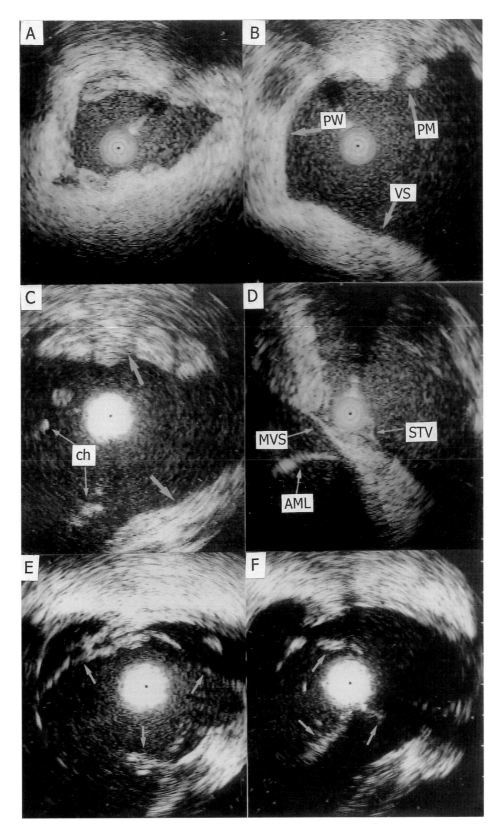

Fig. 5. ICUS images of the normal right ventricle. **A:** outflow level slice. **B:** body level slice. VS: ventricular septum. PW: posterior wall. PM: papillary muscle. **C:** chordal level slice. ch: chordae. **D:** inflow level slice. MVS: membranous ventricular septum. AML: anterior mitral leaflet. STV: septal leaflet of tricuspid valve. **E:** tricuspid leaflets at diastole. **F:** tricuspid leaflets at systole. Arrows: leaflet edges.

of blood is regurgitated from the right ventricle into the right atrium just before complete closure.[6] Probably, this physiological regurgitation is the cause of clinically observed ultrasonographic tricuspid regurgitation.[6]

Cardiac Chambers in Organic Epicardial Coronary Artery Disease

Ventriculographic, Intracardiac Ultrasonographic, Cardioscopic, and Histological Correlations of the Left Ventricle

As a reference, Figs. 6 and 7 show venticulographic, ICUS, and cardioscopic images of a patient with chest pain syndrome. Left ventricular contraction is normal by both ventriculography and ICUS. Cardioscopically, endocardial surface color is nor-

mal reddish brown, trabeculae are not atrophic, and their systolic thickening is obvious, and endocardium and subendocardial myocardium are almost normal by endomyocardial biopsy (Fig. 8A).

Figs. 9 and 10 show images of the left ventricle in a patient with stable angina pectoris due to 2-vessel disease. The left ventricle is normokinetic by ventriculography and ICUS. Myocardial layers are not atrophic, and systolic thickening is preserved by ICUS. Also, trabeculae are not atrophic and systolic thickening is preserved. However, surface color is light brown. Except for slight thickening of the endocardium, no obvious changes are observed histologically (Fig. 8B). These findings indicate existence of mild ischemia without organic myocardial changes in this patient.

Figs. 11 and 12 show images of the left ventricle in a patient with post-infarction angina. The inferior wall is hypokinetic ventriculographically. By ICUS, the same segment is high echoic, and although atrophy is not obvious, systolic thickening is reduced. Cardioscopically, the endocardial surface is diffusely

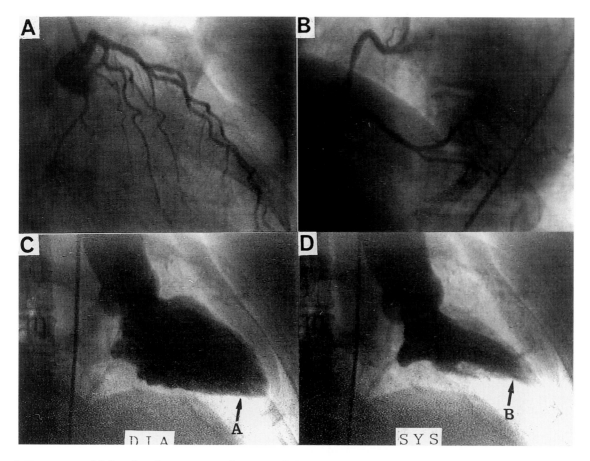

Fig. 6. C.H., 42-year-old female. Chest pain syndrome. **A:** left coronary artery. **B:** right coronary artery. **C:** left ventricle at end-diastole. **D:** left ventricle at end-systole. Arrows A and B: inferior wall observed by cardioscopy and ICUS.

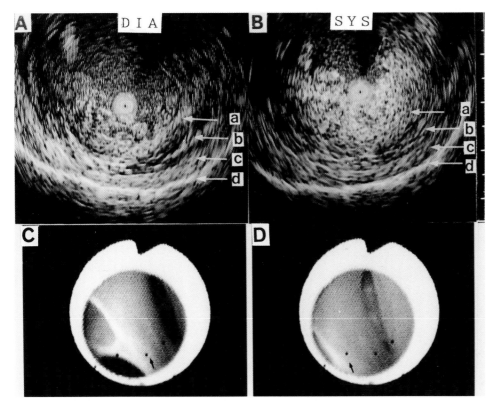

Fig. 7. The same patient as in Fig. 6. **A** and **B**: ICUS images at end-diastole and end-systole, respectively. a: inner oblique layer. b: middle circular layer. c: outer oblique layer. d: pericardium. **C** and **D**: cardioscopic images of the same segment at end-diastole and end-systole, respectively. Arrows: trabeculae.

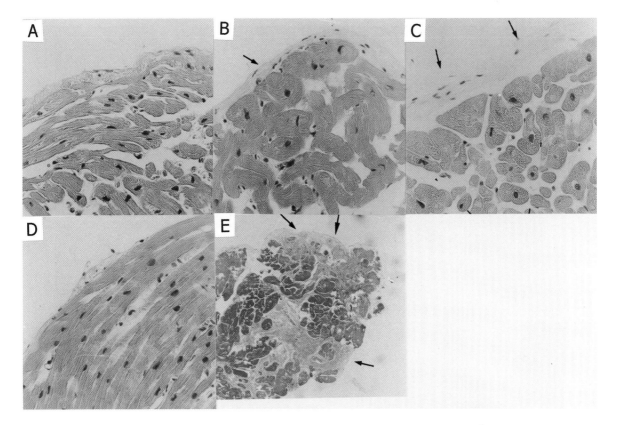

Fig. 8. Biopsy specimens. **A:** the same patient as in Fig. 7. **B:** the same patient as in Fig. 9. **C:** the same patient as in Fig. 11. Thick endocardium and irregular myocytes. **D:** the same patient as in Fig. 13. **E:** the same patient as in Fig. 15. Arrows: fibrosis. HE stain in A to D. Azan stain in E. X400.

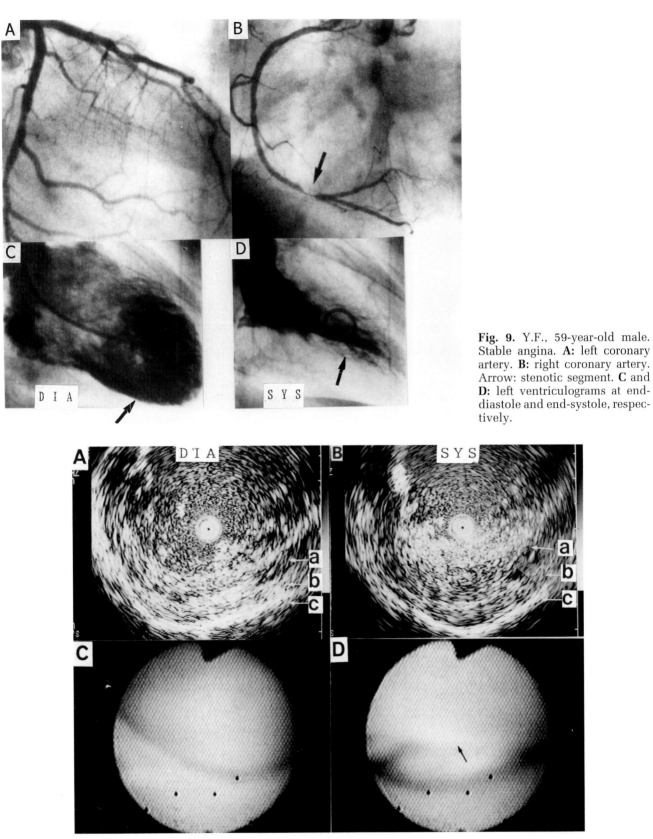

Fig. 9. Y.F., 59-year-old male. Stable angina. **A:** left coronary artery. **B:** right coronary artery. Arrow: stenotic segment. **C** and **D:** left ventriculograms at end-diastole and end-systole, respectively.

Fig. 10. The same patient as in Fig. 9. **A** and **B:** ICUS images at end-diastole and end-systole, respectively. a: inner oblique layer. b: middle circular layer. c: pericardium. **C** and **D:** cardioscopic images at end-diastole and end-systole, respectively. Arrow: trabeculae.

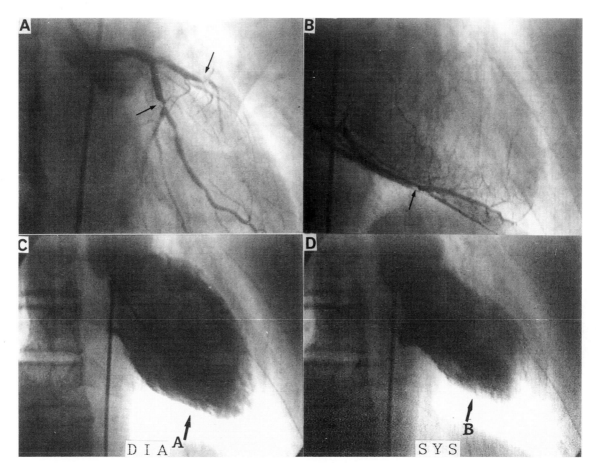

Fig. 11. M.H., 73-year-old male. Old myocardial infarction and stable angina. **A:** left coronary artery. **B:** right coronary artery. Arrows: stenotic segments. **C** and **D:** left ventriculograms at end-diastole and end-systole, respectively. Arrows A and B: observed hypokinetic wall segment.

white, and although trabeculae are not atrophic, their systolic thickening is not obvious as in the case of ICUS. Histologically, the endocardium is thick but myocytes are almost normal (Fig. 8C). The findings indicate hibernating myocardium covered with fibrotic endocardium.

Figs. 13 and 14 show images of the left ventricle in a patient with stable angina due to 3-vessel disease. The inferior wall segment is akinetic by ventriculography. By ICUS, the surface of the trabeculae is high echoic, and although atrophy is not obvious, systolic thickening is not observed. Cardioscopy revealed that the surface is pale and trabeculae are not atrophic, but they are devoid of systolic thickening. Histologically, the endocardium is normal, myocytes are irregular in size, but their loss is not obvious (Fig. 8D). The findings indicate hibernating myocardium.

Figs. 15 and 16 show images of the left ventricle in a patient with an old myocardial infarction. The apical to inferior wall segments are dyskinetic. ICUS revealed thin atrophic and high echoic inner and middle myocardial layers without systolic thickening. Cardioscopy revealed a diffusely white endocardial surface with atrophic trabeculae that are devoid of systolic thickening. Marked myocardial fibrosis is observed histologically (Fig. 8E). The findings indicate advanced fibrosis of the wall.

Tables 1 and 2 show ICUS and cardioscopic classifications of the left ventricle in patients with organic epicardial coronary artery disease and their relation to histological changes.

In our studies, a normal brown and nonatrophic wall was observed preferentially in ventriculographically normokinetic wall segments. A light brown surface and a nonatrophic wall were frequently observed in ventriculographically normokinetic and hypokinetic wall segments. Pale segments without atrophy were frequently observed in ventriculographically akinetic segments. A white surface without atrophy had no relation to ventriculographic wall motion. On the other hand, white-surfaced and atrophic wall segments devoid of systolic thickening

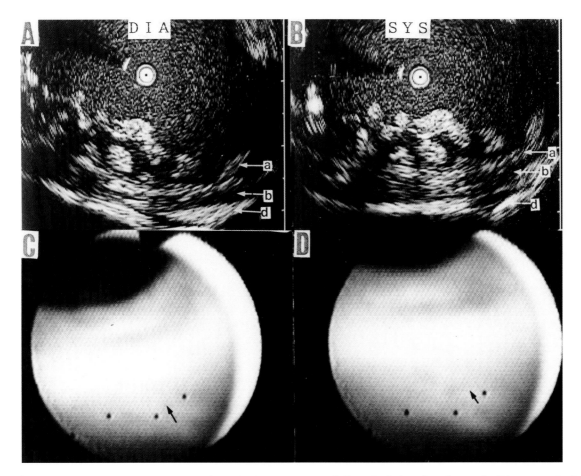

Fig. 12. The same patient as in Fig. 11. **A** and **B:** ICUS images at end-diastole (**A**) and end-systole (**B**), respectively. High echoic inner oblique layer with reduced systolic thickening (a). Systolic thickening of middle circular layer was preserved (b). d: pericardium. **C** and **D:** cardioscopic images of a trabecula (arrow) during diastole and systole. No obvious atrophy but reduced systolic thickening.

were preferentially observed in ventriculographically dyskinetic wall segments. However, endocardial color, ICUS and cardioscopic contraction modality and atrophy had no significant relation to collateral development and severity of the irrigating coronary artery (Fig. 17).

Ventriculographic and Cardioscopic Correlations of the Right Ventricle

Fig. 18 shows ventriculographic and cardioscopic images of the right ventricle in a patient with an old myocardial infarction. The apical wall segment of the right ventricle is akinetic ventriculographically. Cardioscopy revealed a bluish white and akinetic wall with atrophic trabeculae in this akinetic wall segment. Relationships similar to those of the left ventricle were observed between ventriculo-

grams and cardioscopic images of the right ventricle in patients with coronary artery disease.

Cardiac Chambers in Vasospastic Angina Pectoris

The most outstanding cardioscopic changes rather specific to vasospastic angina pectoris are white coloration of the edges of the trabeculae and normal brown color of the free wall. Figs. 19 and 20 show left ventriculographic, ICUS, and cardioscopic changes of the left ventricle in a patient with inducible spasm in the LAD. Ventriculography revealed hypokinetic apical and inferior wall segments. No obvious changes except high echoic endocardium were observed by ICUS. Cardioscopy revealed white trabeculae with a brown free wall.

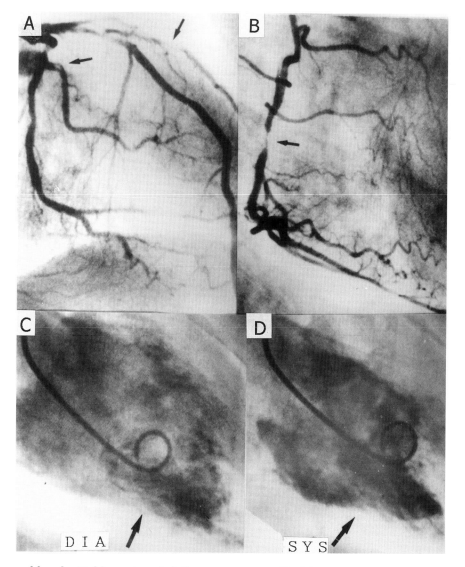

Fig. 13. H.N., 76-year-old male. Stable angina. **A:** left coronary artery. **B:** right coronary artery. Arrows: stenotic segments. **C** and **D:** left ventriculograms at end-diastole and end-systole, respectively. Arrows: akinetic wall segment observed.

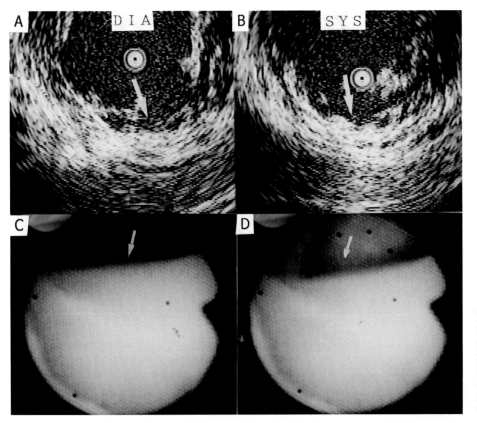

Fig. 14. The same patient as in Fig. 13. **A** and **B:** ICUS images at end-diastole and end-systole, respectively. No obvious systolic thickening. **C** and **D:** cardioscopic images at end-diastole and end-systole, respectively. Pale surface without obvious systolic thickening.

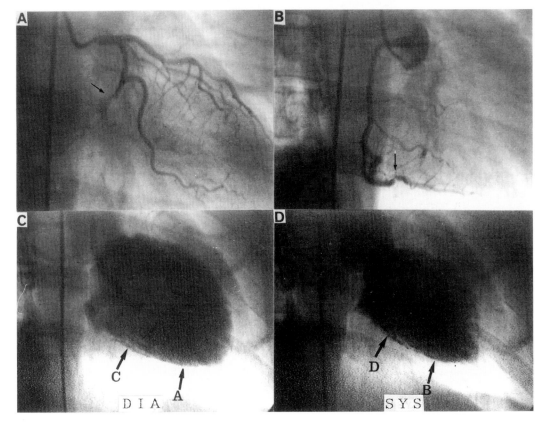

Fig. 15. K.K., 71-year-old male. Old myocardial infarction. **A:** left coronary artery. **B:** right coronary artery. **C** and **D:** left ventriculograms at end-diastole and end-systole, respectively. Arrows A and B: observed dyskinetic wall segment.

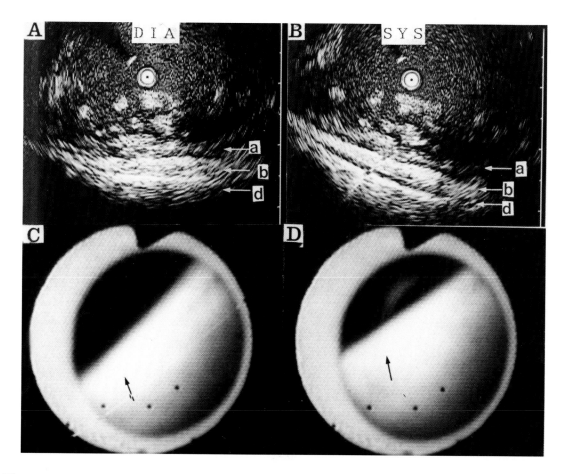

Fig. 16. The same patient as in Fig. 15. **A** and **B:** ICUS images at end-diastole and end-systole, respectively. High echoic, atrophic, and akinetic inner oblique (a) and middle circular (b) layers. d: pericardium. **C** and **D:** cardioscopic images of the same wall segment. Arrows: white, thin and akinetic trabeculae.

Table 1

Intracardiac Ultrasonographic (ICUS) Spectrum of the Left Ventricular Wall in Patients With Coronary Artery Disease

	High Echoic	*Atrophy*	*Systolic Thickening*	*Histological Changes*
Endocardium	+			fibrosis or fibroelastosis
	−			normal
Myocardium	+	+	−	myocyte loss and fibrosis
	−	−	−	hibernation or stunning
	−	−	+	normal

−: absent. +: present.

Table 2
Cardioscopic Spectrum of the Ventricle in Patients With Coronary Artery Disease

Endocardial Color	Atrophic Trabeculae	Systolic Thickening	Blood Flow	Histological Changes Endocardium	Myocardium
Brown	−	−	−	−	−
Light brown	−	− or reduced	reduced	−	−
Pale	−	−	severely reduced	−	− or +
White	−	− or reduced	− or reduced	+	− or +
	+	−	−	+	+
Yellow				fibroelastosis	
Pink, red, or purplish red				reactive hyperemia or drug effects	

nor: normal. −: absent. +: present.

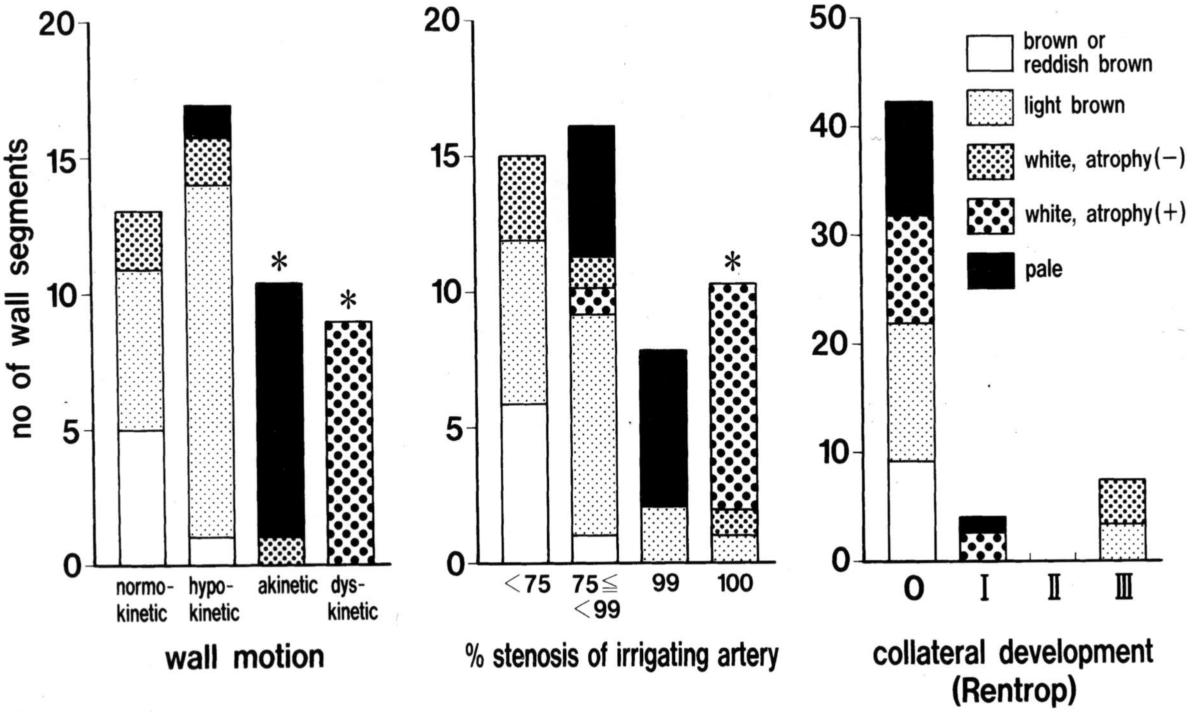

Fig. 17. Relations of endocardial color of the left ventricle to wall motion, severity of stenosis of the irrigating coronary artery, and collateral development. * P < 0.05.

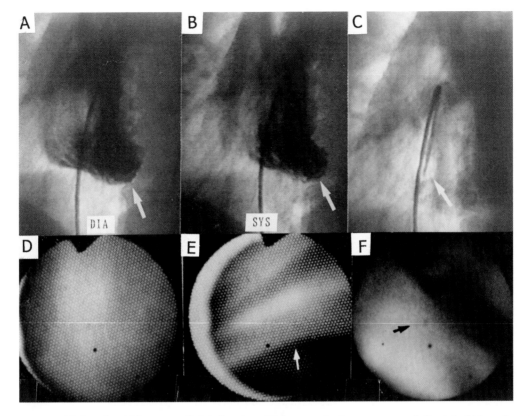

Fig. 18. C.M., 63-year-old female. Old myocardial infarction. Right ventriculograms at end-diastole (**A**), end-systole (**B**) and during cardioscopic observation (**C**). Arrows in A, B: correspond to F. Arrow in C: cardioscope. Cardioscopic images of normokinetic posterobasal wall segment (**D**), hypokinetic anteroapical wall segment (**E**), and akinetic apical wall segment (**F**).

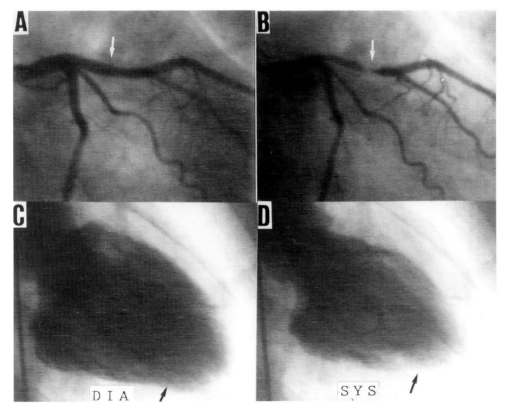

Fig. 19. J.H., 53-year-old female. Vasospastic angina. **A** and **B**: coronary angiograms showing segmental spasm induced by intracoronary injection of ergonovine maleate. **C** and **D**: left ventriculograms at end-diastole and end-systole, respectively. Arrows: observed hypokinetic inferior wall segment.

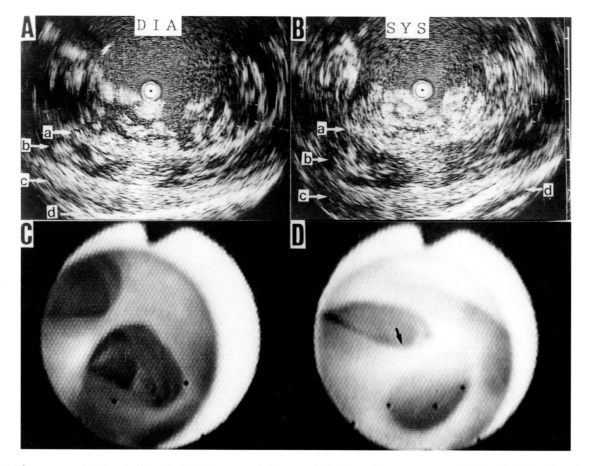

Fig. 20. The same patient as in Fig. 19. ICUS images of the same inferior wall segment at end-diastole (**A**) and end-systole (**B**), respectively. Systolic thickening of inner oblique (a) and middle circular (b) layers. c: outer oblique layer. d: pericardium. **C** and **D**: cardioscopic images at end-diastole and end-systole. Arrow in D: white trabecula.

Biopsy of the trabeculae revealed fibrosis of the trabecular edges (Fig. 21). Probably, transient but severe and recurrent myocardial ischemia resulted in myocyte degeneration and fibrosis in the edges that are most susceptible to ischemia. These histological changes may contribute to relaxation impairment of the left ventricle in patients with this category of coronary artery disease.

Inflammatory cells are increased in the majority of patients with this category of disease irrespective of segmental and diffuse spasm, and therefore they may be misdiagnosed as myocarditis. It is well known that inflammatory cell infiltration occurs in response to severe myocardial ischemia. Therefore, increased inflammatory cells may mean that severe myocardial ischemia recently occurred.

Since left ventricular damages in patients with vasospastic angina differ from patient to patient, we developed a cardioscopic and histological scoring system of the left ventricle for patient-to-patient comparison and for follow-up study (Tables 3 and 4).

Cardiac Chambers in Microvessel Disease

We saw 7 patients with microvessel disease. Left ventricular contraction was almost normal in all 7. However, the apical wall segment was diffusely light brown in 2 and white and light brown speckled in 5 patients. Biopsy revealed thick-walled arterioles and spotty fibrosis in all (Fig. 22).

Octopus Pod-Like Cardiomyopathy

Reversible contraction disturbance is caused by subarachnoid hemorrhage, catecholamines (catecholamine cardiomyopathy or catecholamine myocarditis), emotional stress, traumatic asphyxia, and noncardiac surgery in elderly patients.[9–13] There is a new entity of cardiomyopathy characterized by a

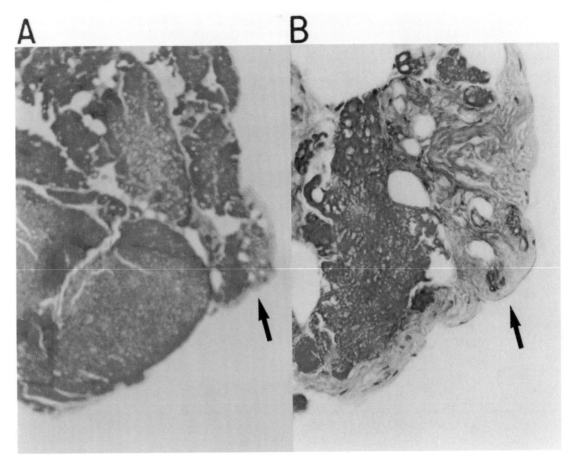

Fig. 21. Biopsy specimen. **A:** ×100. **B:** ×400. Arrows: fibrotic trabecular edge. Azan stain.

Table 3
**Cardioscopic Scoring of the Ventricle
in Patients With Vasospastic Angina**

1. Free wall					
Color	brown	light brown	white and brown speckled	white	yellow
Score	*0*	*1*	*2*	*3*	*3*
2. Trabeculae					
a) White portion (%)	none	<25	25 ≤ <50	50≤ <75	75 ≤
Score	*0*	*1*	*2*	*3*	*4*
b) Atrophy	Absent	Present			
Score	*0*	*1*			
c) Systolic thickening	Present	Absent			
Score	*0*	*1*			

Table 4
Biopsy Scoring of the Left Ventricle in Patients With Vasospastic Angina

1. Mononuclear cell infiltration (Inflammation) No of cells					
/f at ×200	<5	5≤ <10	10≤ < 20	20≤ <50	50≤
Score	*0*	*1*	*2*	*3*	*4*
2. Interstitial fibrosis					
% area	<5	5≤ <15	15≤ < 25	25≤ <50	50≤
Score	*0*	*1*	*2*	*3*	*4*
3. Interstitial edema	Absent	Present			
Score	*0*	*1*			
4. Myocytes	Absent	Present			
Hypertrophy	0	1			
Vacuolization	0	1			
Myofilament loss	0	1			
Myocyte loss	0	1			
Contraction band Necrosis	0	1			
5. Endocardial fibrosis					
Thickness (μm)	<25	25≤ <50	50≤ <100	100≤	
Score	*1*	*2*	*3*	*4*	
6. Endocardial edema	Absent	Present			
Score	*0*	*1*			

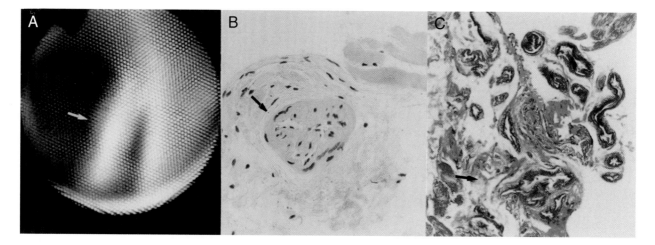

Fig. 22. I.T., 40-year-old male. Stable angina due to microvessel disease. **A:** white trabeculae in the apical wall segment. **B:** thick-walled arteriole (arrow) surrounded by fibrotic tissues (arrow). HE stain. ×400. **C:** marked fibrosis around the vessels (arrow). TPHA stain. ×400.

queer feature of the left ventriculogram. This cardiomyopathy exhibits an octopus pod-like left ventricle ventriculographically, due to hypo- to dyskinetic anteroapical wall and hyperkinetic basal wall. The majority of patients of this category are elderly females. Chest pain or congestive heart failure occurs abruptly associated with elevation of the ST segment of the electrocardiogram, sometimes preceded by severe emotional stress. Coronary angiograms taken during ST elevation are normal. Coronary spasm is induced in a certain group of the patients. Contraction disturbance is rapidly improved within a few

days to a few weeks. In the acute phase, focal myocyte loss and inflammatory cell infiltration are frequently observed. Focal fibrosis is observed not only in the later phase but also in the acute phase.[13]

An elderly female was admitted to our hospital due to dyspnea that occurred a few hours after the sudden death of her daughter. The ST segment of the electrocardiogram was elevated in II, III, aVF, and V_{2-6}. CK-MB was not elevated. Left ventriculograms obtained 6 hours after the onset of the attack revealed a typical octopus pod-like configuration. Coronary angiograms were normal. Cardioscopy of

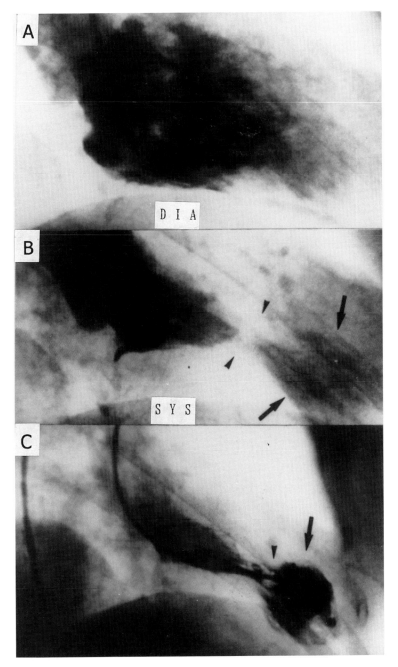

Fig. 23. T.K., 78-year-old female. Octopus pod-like cardiomyopathy. Left ventriculograms at end-diastole (**A**) and end-systole (**B**) and during cardioscopic observation of dyskinetic apical wall segment (**C**) 6 hours after the onset of the attack. Arrow in B: dyskinetic apical wall segment. Arrowhead: hyperkinetic middle wall segment. Arrow in C: guiding balloon catheter.

the apical segment showed a yellowish brown surface. Biopsy revealed focal myocyte lysis and focal mononuclear cell infiltration but not contraction band necrosis. Repeated ventriculograms obtained 1 month later revealed improved left ventricular contraction. Coronary spasm was induced by intracoronary administration of acetylcholine. Cardioscopy showed a speckled yellowish brown and white endocardial surface. Biopsy revealed focal fibrosis (Figs. 23–26).

Myocardial stunning after coronary spasm, myocardial intoxication due to excessive outflow of catecholamine induced by emotional stress, and acute myocarditis are postulated as the possible causative mechanisms of this category of disease. However, exact mechanisms are not known. Coronary spasm was considered to be the major causative factor at least in this patient. However, yellowish brown discoloration of the left ventricle suggested preceding endocardiomyocardial changes.

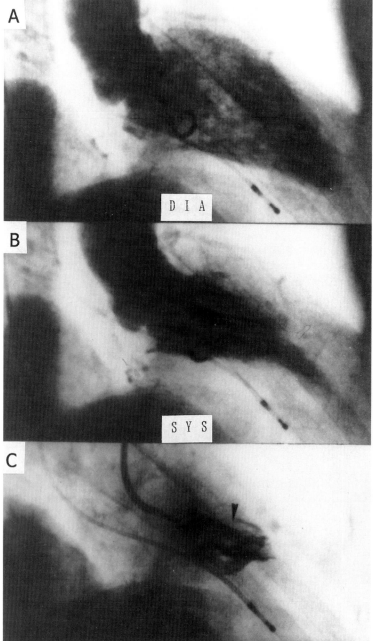

Fig. 24. The same patient as in Fig. 23. Ventriculograms at end-diastole (**A**) and end-systole (**B**) and during cardioscopic observation (**C**) taken 1 month later. Arrow in C: guiding balloon catheter.

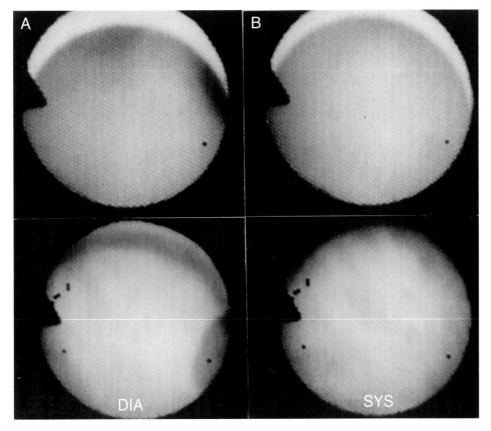

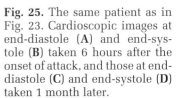

Fig. 25. The same patient as in Fig. 23. Cardioscopic images at end-diastole (**A**) and end-systole (**B**) taken 6 hours after the onset of attack, and those at end-diastole (**C**) and end-systole (**D**) taken 1 month later.

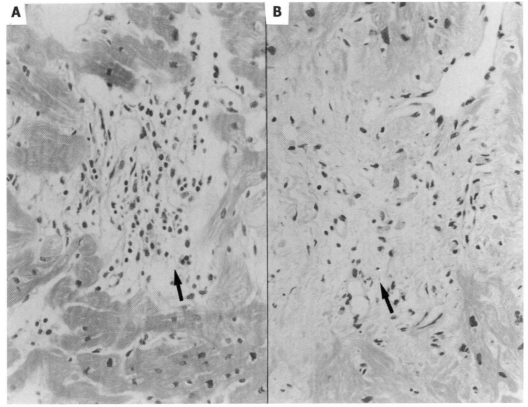

Fig. 26. Biopsy specimens. **A:** 6 hours after the onset of attack. Focal loss of myocytes, interstitial edema, and mononuclear cell infiltration. **B:** 1 month later. Focal fibrosis and mononuclear cell infiltration. HE stain. ×400.

References

1. Uchida Y: Atlas of Cardioangioscopy. Medical View Co., Tokyo, 1997.
2. Uchida Y, Tomaru T, Nakamura F, et al: Percutaneous fiberoptic angioscopy of the left ventricle. Jpn Heart J 32:455–471, 1991.
3. Uchida Y, Oshima T, Yoshihara F, et al: Percutaneous fiberoptic angioscopy of cardiac valves. Am Heart J 121:1791–1798, 1991.
4. Uchida Y, Hirose J, Oshima T, et al: Discrimination of left ventricular myocardial layers by intracardiac ultrasound in patients with ischemic heart disease. Circulation 98(Suppl):I-533, 1997.
5. Uchida Y: Percutaneous angioscopy of cardiac chambers and valves. In: Progress in Cardiology. Zipes D (ed). Lea & Febiger, Philadelphia, 1991, pp 163–192.
6. Uchida Y, Oshima T, Shibuya I: Percutaneous angioscopy of the right side of the heart in humans. Cardiovasc World Report 1:13–17, 1988.
7. Uchida Y, Tomaru T, Kato S: Percutaneous pulmonary angioscopy using a balloon guiding catheter. Clin Cardiol 11:143–148, 1988.
8. Uchida Y, Oshima T, Hirose J, et al: Angioscopic detection of residual pulmonary thrombi in the differential diagnosis of pulmonary embolism. Am Heart J 130:854–859, 1995.
9. Sakamoto H: Abnormal Q wave, ST elevation, T-wave inversion, and widespread focal myocytolysis associated with subarachnoid hemorrhage. Jpn Circulat J 60:254–257, 1996.
10. Furtstaci A, Leoperifido F, Gentiloni N: Catecholamine-induced cardiomyopathy in multiple endocrine neoplasia: A histologic, ultrastructural, and biochemical study. Chest 99:382–385, 1991.
11. Cebelin MS, Hirsch CS: Human stress cardiomyopathy: Myocardial lesions in victims of homicidal assault without internal injuries. Human Pathol 11:123–132, 1980.
12. Kawai S: TAKOTSUBO cardiomyopathy: Reversible round bottom flask-like asynergy of the left ventricle. Therap Res 20:86–93, 1999 (in Japanese).
13. Satoh M, Tateishi H, Uchida T, et al: Pod-like left ventricle due to stunned myocardium induced by multivessel spasm. In: Clinical Myocyte Lesions. Kodama K, Hori S (eds). Kagaku Hyouron Co., Tokyo, 1990, pp 56–64 (in Japanese).

Chapter 23

Cardioscopic Images of the Left Ventricle in Different Heart Diseases for Differential Diagnosis

In order to differentiate ischemic heart disease from other categories of heart disease, we should be familiar with typical cardioscopic images of various categories of heart disease.

Fig. 1 shows representative examples of acute myocarditis, chronic active myocarditis, idiopathic dilated cardiomyopathy, idiopathic hypertrophic cardiomyopathy, rheumatic endomyocarditis, and metabolic heart disease.[1-3] Differentiation of ischemic heart disease from rheumatic heart disease is sometimes difficult because endomyocardial fibrosis occurs in both. However, typical changes in cardiac valves and chordae greatly contribute to differential diagnosis.

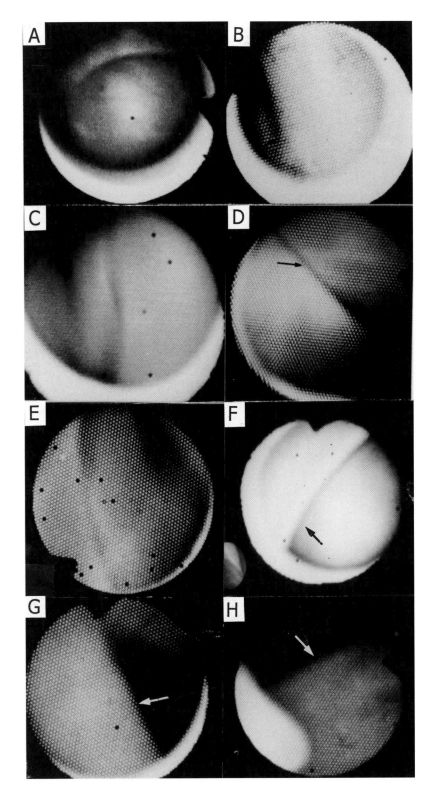

Fig. 1. Endocardial surface of the left ventricle in various categories of heart disease. **A:** red endocardial surface in idiopathic acute myocarditis. **B:** milky white surface due to inflammatory endocardial edema in acute myocarditis. **C:** yellowish brown endocardial surface due to endocardial fibroelastosis in chronic inactive myocarditis. **D:** thick, white trabeculae in idiopathic hypertrophic cardiomyopathy. **E:** white and brown speckled endocardial surface with atrophic trabeculae in idiopathic dilated cardiomyopathy. **F:** diffusely white endocardial surface due to fibrosis and atrophic trabeculae in idiopathic dilated cardiomyopathy. **G:** purplish red endocardial surface in chronic active myocarditis. **H:** lined or spotty deposition of amyloid in cardiac amyloidosis.

References

1. Uchida Y, Nakamura F, Oshima T, et al: Percutaneous fiberoptic angioscopy of the left ventricle in patients with dilated cardiomyopathy and acute myocarditis. Am Heart J 120:677–687, 1990.
2. Uchida Y, Oshima T, Yoshihara F, et al: Percutaneous fiberoptic angioscopy of cardiac valves. Am Heart J 121:1791–1798, 1991.
3. Uchida Y: Atlas of Cardioangioscopy. Medical View Co., Tokyo, 1997.

Chapter 24

Subendocardial Microvessels

Microvessels ranging from 20 to 100 μm in diameter are frequently observed in both normal and diseased left ventricles. They are exposed in the cavity (Fig. 1A) or exist beneath the endocardium (Fig. 1B).[1] They are straight or hemangiomatous (Fig. 1C, D). The color of the blood in the vessels is either red or purple. Red indicates that the vessels are arterial and purple indicates that the vessels are venous in nature (Fig. 1D).

We found 38 vessels in 236 patients who underwent cardioscopy of the left ventricle. The vessels were found in 25% of patients with old myocardial infarction and in 10.5% of patients with angina. The majority of the vessels were located beneath the endocardium and were arterial in nature (Table 1). A certain group of the vessels beneath the endocardium collapsed during systole (Fig. 2), while those exposed in the cavity did not. Their responses to nitroglycerin were examined. Collapse followed by dilatation was observed in response to the agent but not in all. The reason for their differential response to cardiac contraction and vasodilators remains to be elucidated.

Examination of their responses to various stresses including medical, interventional, and surgical therapies may reveal hitherto unanswered phenomena of microcirculation in the myocardium.

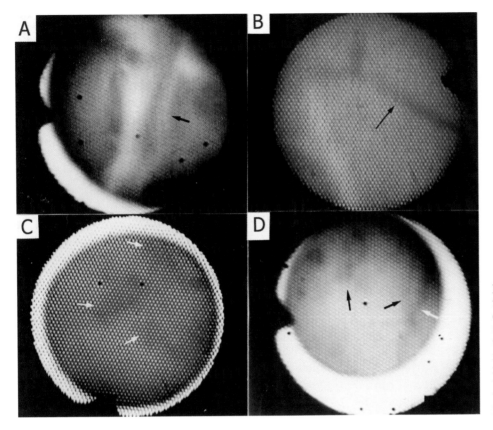

Fig. 1. Microvessels observed in the left ventricle. **A:** arterial vessel exposed in the ventricular cavity (arrow). **B:** arterial vessel beneath the endocardium (arrow). **C:** hemangiomatous arterial vessels (arrows). **D:** hemangiomatous venous vessels (arrowhead). Black arrows: venous vessel. White arrow: arterial vessel.

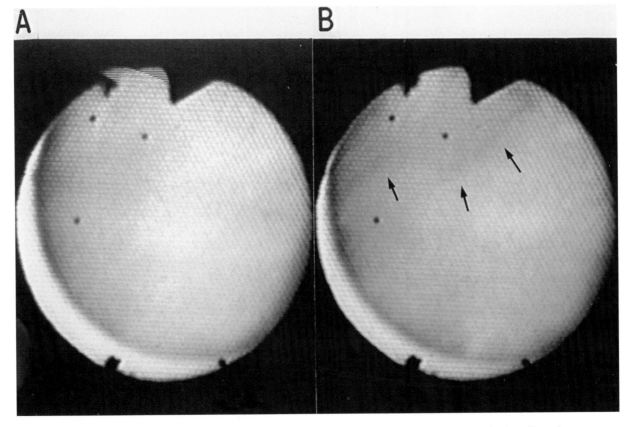

Fig. 2. Subendocardial microvessel. **A:** collapse during systole. **B:** reappearance during diastole.

Table 1
Microvessels Observed in the Left Ventricle

A. Microvessels in different categories of heart disease

Disease	No of patients	Microvessels observed (%)
OMI	64	16 (25.0)
AP	57	6 (10.5)
HCM	11	1 (9.2)
DCM	10	3 (30.0)
MC	89	11 (12.3)
CP	5	1 (16.1)
Total	236	38 (16.1)

OMI: old myocardial infarction. AP: angina pectoris. HCM: idiopathic hypertrophic cardiomyopathy. DCM: idiopathic dilated cardiomyopathy. MC: myocarditis. CP: chest pain syndrome.

B. Locations of microvessels

Total	Beneath endocardium	Exposed in cavity	On thrombus
38	31	5	2

C. Classification of microvessels

Total	arterial	venous
38	30	8

D. Responses to myocardial contraction

	Systolic collapse		
	Total	Present	Absent
Arterial	30	12	18
Venous	8	3	5

E. Responses to nitroglycerin

Total	Collapse followed by dilatation	No change
5	3	2

References

1. Uchida Y: Atlas of Cardioangioscopy. Medical View Co., Tokyo, 1997.

2. Uchida Y, Kawai K, Ohsawa H, et al: Direct visualization of subendocardial microvessels by percutaneous cardioscopy. Circulation 98(Suppl):I-489, 1998.

Chapter 25

Thrombus in the Cardiac Chambers

Ischemic heart disease is not infrequently associated with thrombus on the ventricular endocardium.[1,2] It is generally believed that blood stagnation due to contraction disturbance results in thrombus formation.

Fig. 1 shows a patient with old myocardial infarction in whom a large globular mass suggesting thrombus was found in the apical segment of the left ventricle by transthoracic echocardiography. Left ventriculography revealed a globular mass in the dyskinetic apical segment due to total occlusion of the LAD. A cardioscope was carefully introduced into the left ventricle so as not to touch the mass. By infusing saline, it was slowly advanced toward the mass and a red thrombus was clearly observed. This is the standard cardioscopic technique for observation of a thrombus in the heart. Although the attack occurred more than 1 month earlier, the thrombus was red, suggesting that thrombosis continued while autolysis was occurring. Three months after warfarin therapy, the mass was not detected by echocardiography and left ventriculography. Cardioscopy re-vealed yellow spots on the endocardium, suggesting organized residual thrombus. Cardioscopically, ventricular thrombi are classified by shape into globular (protruded) and mural (lined), and by color into red, white, and yellow. Yellow and white thrombi frequently glistened, reflecting illumination (Fig. 2).

Table 1 summarizes the incidence of ventricular thrombi not only in patients with ischemic heart disease but also in patients with other categories of heart disease. It was revealed that the incidence of thrombi detected by cardioscopy is 18.6% in patients with myocardial infarction and 12.3% in angina pectoris. Since cardioscopic observation was performed in very small portions of the ventricle, the exact incidence may be far higher.

The thrombi were found not only in the wall segments with obvious contraction disturbance but also in those without, suggesting that blood turbulence due to contraction disturbance is not the sole cause of thrombosis. Probably, endocardial damage due to ischemia may also contribute to thrombogenesis as in vessels.

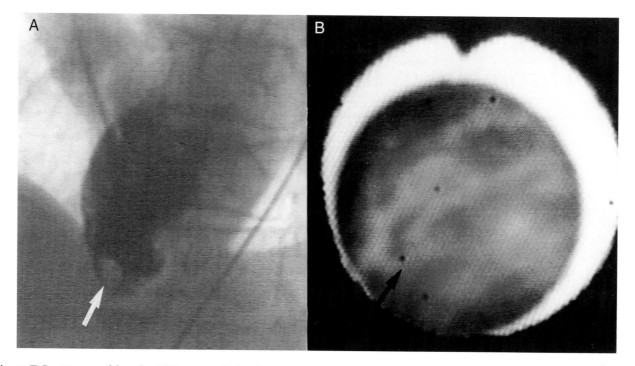

Fig. 1. T.O., 57-year-old male. Old myocardial infarction. **A:** Left ventriculogram at LAO. Arrow: a negative shadow suggesting thrombus. **B:** red thrombus corresponding to the shadow in A (arrow).

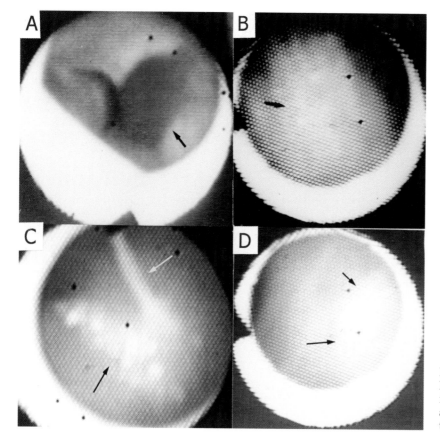

Fig. 2. Color of thrombi. **A:** red thrombus. **B:** glistening yellow thrombus. **C:** glistening white thrombus (black arrow). White arrow: chorda. **D:** nonglistening white thrombus.

Table 1
Ventricular Thrombus in Different Categories of Heart Disease

Disease	No. of Patients	Incidence (%)	Configuration		In Diseased Wall Segment	Detected by	
			Mural	Globular		UCG	VG
1. Left Ventricle							
Myocardial infarction	64	12 (18.6)	9	3	7	3	2
Angina pectoris	57	7 (12.3)	7	0	1	0	0
Myocarditis	89	28 (31.9)	26	2	11	2	2
Rheumatic valvular disease	6	2 (33.3)	2	0	0	0	0
2. Right Ventricle							
Myocardial infarction	10	2 (20.0)	1	1	2	0	0
Pacemaker lead	5	3 (60.0)	2	1	0	1	0

UCG: ultrasonic echocardiography. VG: ventriculography.

References

1. Uchida Y: Atlas of Cardioangioscopy. Medical View Co., Tokyo, 1997.
2. Oshima T, Hirose J, Sasaki M, et al: Detection of mural thrombus of the left ventricle by percutaneous cardioscopy. Circulation 90(Suppl 4-II):I-450, 1994.

Chapter 26

Dye Image Cardioscopy for Detection of Endocardial Cell Damage and Evaluation of Myocardial Blood Flow

Discrimination of Endocardial Cell Damage

Recent cardioscopic examinations of the left ventricle revealed frequent existence of mural thrombi in the left ventricle not only in patients with myocardial diseases but also in patients with ischemic heart disease and without obvious contraction disturbance.[1] This fact indicates that blood stagnation due to contraction disturbance is not the sole cause of thrombus formation. There is a possibility that endocardial cell damage due to reduction of blood supply through the coronary artery results in thrombus formation.

Discrimination of endocardial cell damage is beyond conventional cardioscopy. We found that Evans blue dye, which selectively stains damaged vascular endothelial cells of vessels,[2] also selectively stains endocardial cells. Therefore, we applied dye image cardioscopy for discrimination of endocardial cell damage.

Fig. 1 shows white trabecular edges in a patient with vasospastic angina pectoris. The edges were stained in blue with Evans blue, indicating that the endocardial cells on the edges were damaged. Probably, transient but severe ischemia due to vasospasm resulted in not only myocardial but also endocardial cell damage.

As summarized in Table 1, endocardial damage was observed with high frequency not only in myocardial but also in coronary artery disease. This damage, which was not detectable by other means, may be the source of cerebral thromboembolism in patients without demonstrable sources.[3]

Evaluation of Myocardial Blood Flow

Dye image cardioscopy is also useful for identification of regional myocardial blood flow. During observation of a wall segment, a selective bolus injection of 1 mL of 2% Evans blue solution into the irrigating coronary artery results in staining of the wall segment when the artery is patent (Fig. 2) but not when the artery is obstructed. This method can be used for visual identification of subendocardial myocardial blood flow changes.

235

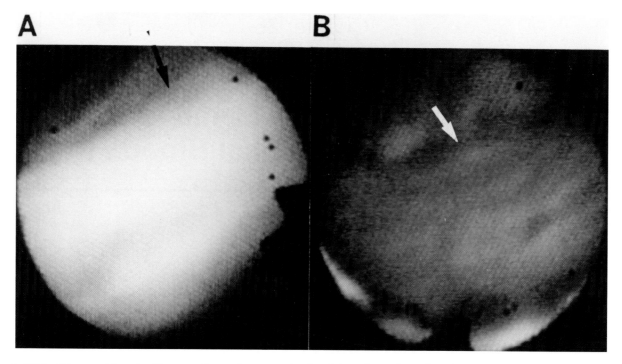

Fig. 1. Y.M., 66-year-old male. Vasospastic angina pectoris. **A:** white edges of a trabeculae in the left ventricle (arrow). **B:** the same edge was stained with Evans blue (arrow).

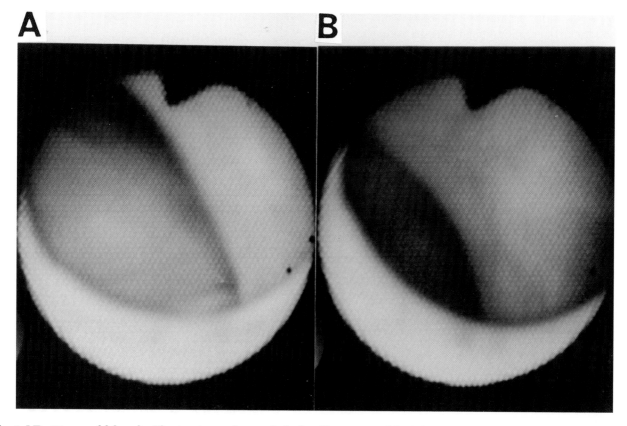

Fig. 2. I.T., 45-year-old female. Chest pain syndrome. Apical wall segment of the left ventricle before (**A**) and 5 minutes after the injection of 1 mL of 2% Evans blue into the LAD (**B**). Diffusely stained portion indicates preserved myocardial blood flow.

Table 1
Endocardial Staining With Evans Blue

Disease	No. of Patients	Stained
Angina pectoris	16	10 (63%)
Old myocardial infarction	10	10 (100%)
Dilated cardiomyopathy	11	8 (73%)
Chest pain syndrome	8	3 (38%)

References

1. Uchida Y: Atlas of Cardioangioscopy. Medical View Co., Tokyo, 1997.
2. Uchida Y, Nakamura F, Morita T: Observation of atherosclerotic plaques by an intravascular microscope in patients with arteriosclerosis obliterans. Am Heart J 130:1114–1117, 1995.
3. Rocotta JJ, Faggioli GL, Castilone A, et al: Risk factors for stroke after cardiac surgery: Buffalo Cardiac-Cerebral Study Group. J Vasc Surg 21:359–364, 1995.

Chapter 27

Fluorescent Image Cardioscopy for Assessment of Regional Myocardial Blood Flow

Fluorescein isothiocyanate conjugated (FITC) generates fluorescence at 520 nm when excited by 490 nm, and it is routinely used for detection of retinal artery microaneuryms in patients with diabetes mellitus.[1] When injected into a vessel, this substance is diffused through the vascular wall into the tissues. Therefore, existence of fluorescence in the tissue indicates existence of blood flow supplied by the vessel.

Fig. 1 shows a fluorescent image of the left ventricle obtained after the injection of 1 mL of 1% FITC into the right coronary artery in a patient with angina pectoris. Both the free wall and the trabeculae exhibited fluorescence. Trabeculae exhibited stronger fluorescence than the free wall, suggesting that blood flow was more dominant in the former. Since it is a very sensitive method, it can be used for evaluation of regional subendocardial myocardial blood flow in patients with ischemic heart disease and for evaluation of medical, interventional, and surgical therapies.

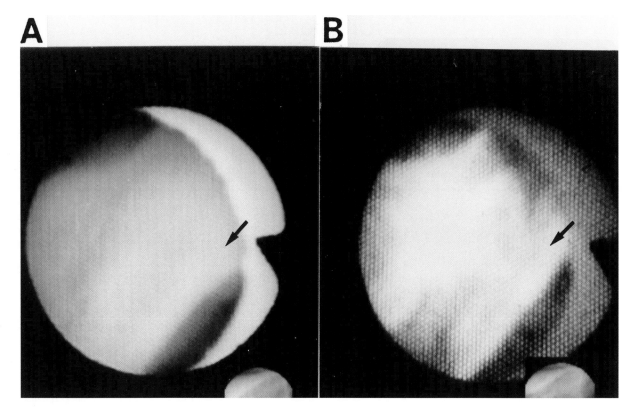

Fig. 1. U.R., 71-year-old male. Angina pectoris. **A:** conventional cardioscopic appearance of the inferior wall. **B:** fluorescence image of the same portion 1 minute after selective injection of 1 mL of 1% FITC into the right coronary artery.

Reference

1. Brubaker RF: Measurement of fluorescein-binding in human plasma using fluorescein polarization. Arch Ophthalmol 100:625–630, 1982.

Chapter 28

Cardioscopic Evaluation of Myocardial Blood Flow Restoration Induced by Medical, Interventional, and Surgical Therapies

Medical Therapy

Intravenous injection of nitroglycerin (200 μg) was performed in patients with different endocardial colors. Fig. 1 shows pale endocardial color, which changed to pink 3 minutes after 200 μg nitroglycerin. Pink indicates increased arterial blood in the subendocardial myocardial layers. Also, contraction was improved in this patient. Fig. 2 also shows pale endocardial color that changed to purplish red, indicating increased venous blood. It is likely that shifting of the blood from subepicardial layers to subendocardial layers occurred due to a decrease in the ratio of diastolic pressure time index/tension time index.[1] In the majority of wall segments that exhibited brown and light brown, the color changed to reddish brown or pink, indicating increased or restored blood flow. Interestingly, in the majority of pale wall segments, the color changed to either pink or purplish red. Furthermore, contraction was restored (Table 1). Biopsy revealed insignificant changes in the majority of the wall segments, indicating that a pale wall segment contains hibernating myocardium.

A certain group of white wall segments also responded to nitroglycerin. Fig. 3 shows a white wall segment. Following nitroglycerin, a pink layer was seen through the white layer, indicating that the myocardial blood flow beneath the fibrotic endocardium was restored. Changes in hemodynamic parameters, except control of left ventricular systolic pressure, had no relation to those in wall color changes (Fig. 4). Probably, multifactors such as severity of myocardial changes and stenoses of the irrigating artery, collateral developments, and hemodynamic changes influence nitroglycerin-induced changes in subendocardial myocardial blood flow.

Interventional Therapy

In a small number of patients, cardioscopy of the same wall segments was performed before and immediately after coronary interventions. It was revealed that wall color was also improved by coronary interventions (Table 1).

Angiogenic Therapy

According to our study, about 15% of patients with ischemic heart disease are not candidates for interventional and surgical therapies. However, there are at present no other curative modalities for them.[2] Myocardial salvage by new formation of blood vessels by either angiogenesis or vasculogenesis (angiogenic therapy) is one promising therapeutic modality for these patients.

In 1992, we found that a growth factor with basic fibroblast growth factor (bFGF) can salvage infarcted myocardium in an experimental canine model of acute myocardial infarction.[3–5] Since then, many investigators have attempted to establish angiogenic therapy for patients.

Possible candidates for angiogenic therapy are those with ischemic heart disease and myocardial disease such as idiopathic dilated cardiomyopathy. Therefore, we have been attempting this therapy in patients with these categories of heart disease and peripheral atherosclerotic disease.[6]

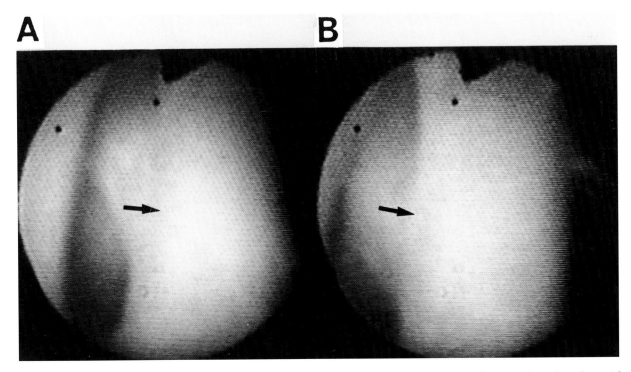

Fig. 1. K.S., 58-year-old female. Stable angina pectoris. Apical segment of the left ventricle. **A:** pale trabeculae without atrophy before nitroglycerin. **B:** 3 minutes after intravenous injection of 200 μg nitroglycerin. Note the pink color.

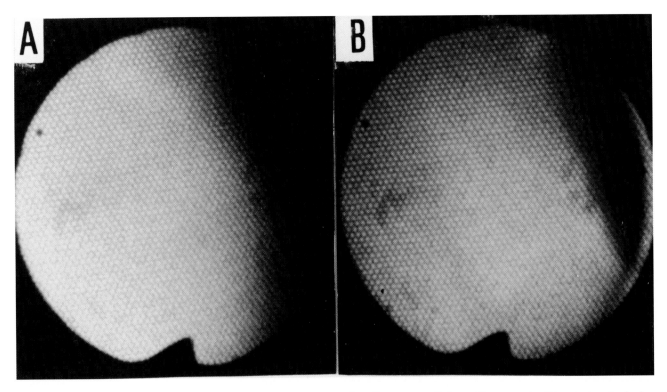

Fig. 2. A.S., 56-year-old male. Old myocardial infarction. Lateral wall segment. Pale wall segment without atrophy before (**A**), changed to purplish red (**B**) 3 minutes after 200 μg nitroglycerin.

Table 1
Effects of Nitroglycerin and Coronary Interventions on Left Ventricular Endocardial Coloration

			Color		
No. of segments examined	*Brown* *4*	*Light Brown* *4*	*Pale* *10*	*White* *12* *atrophy (−)* *3*	*atrophy (+)* *9*
1. Atrophic trabeculae					9
2. Wall motion					
Normokinetic	4				
Hypokinetic		4	1	2	
Akinetic			9	1	1
Dyskinetic					8
3. Stenosis of irrigating artery (%)					
75>	4	2		1	
75< <99		2	4	1	1
99			6	1	1
100					7
4. Nitroglycerin (200 μg)					
Improved color	4	4	9	2	1
Improved contraction		3	8	2	
5. Biopsy					
Myocyte loss			1	1	9
Myocardial fibrosis		1	2	1	9
Endocardial fibrosis			1	3	9
6. Response to POBA					
Underwent POBA		2	6	2	4
Improved color		2	6	1	4
Improved contraction		2	6	1	

POBA: plain old balloon angioplasty.

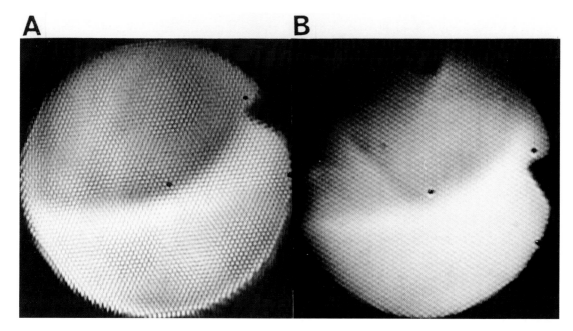

Fig. 3. K.Y., 70-year-old male. Old myocardial infarction. Apical segment. **A:** white trabeculae. **B:** subendocardial layers with pink coloration was seen through the white layer (fibrotic endocardium proven by biopsy) 3 minutes after 200 μg nitroglycerin.

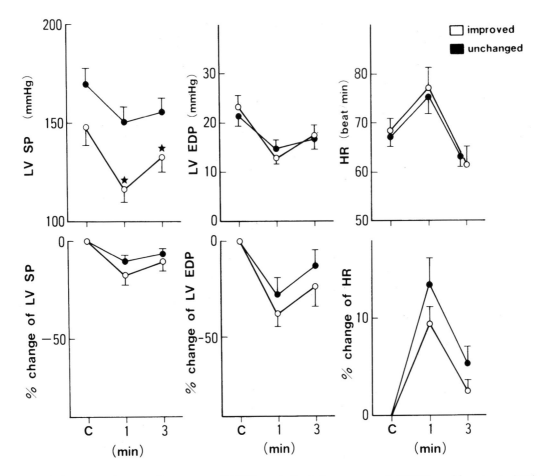

Fig. 4. Changes in left ventricular systolic pressure (LVSP), end-diastolic pressure (LVEDP), and heart rate (HR) induced by intravenous injection of 200 μg nitroglycerin and their relation to endocardial coloration. **C:** before nitroglycerin.

Fig. 5 shows left ventriculograms before and 3 months after selective intracoronary bolus injection of 100 μg bFGF, which was performed 2 years after medical therapy in a patient with idiopathic dilated cardiomyopathy. After 3 months, contraction of apical to posterior wall segments was much improved. Although angiography did not show any obvious increase in the number of coronary vessels,

the endocardial color changed from pale to pink, suggesting blood flow restoration (Fig. 6). In addition, biopsy revealed increased capillaries and arterioles (Figs. 7, 8). This fact indicates that angiogenic therapy is also effective in a certain group of patients with dilated cardiomyopathy and that cardioscopy is useful for evaluation of angiogenic therapy.

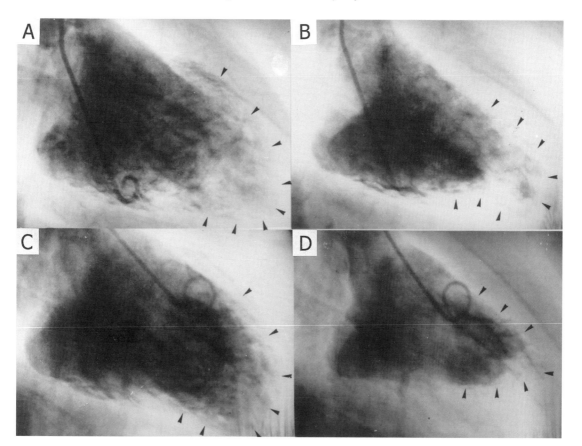

Fig. 5. K.O., 36-year-old male. Idiopathic dilated cardiomyopathy. Left ventriculograms at end-diastole (**A**) and end-systole (**B**) before, and those at end-diastole (**C**) and end-systole (**D**) 3 months after the injection of 100 µg human recombinant bFGF into the right coronary artery.

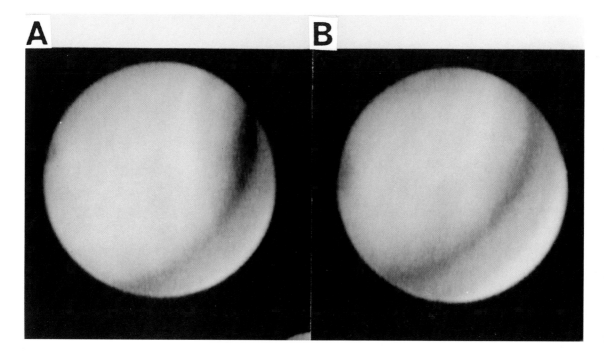

Fig. 6. The same patient as in Fig. 5. Cardioscopic images during diastole (**A**) and systole (**B**) of posterior wall segment before treatment.

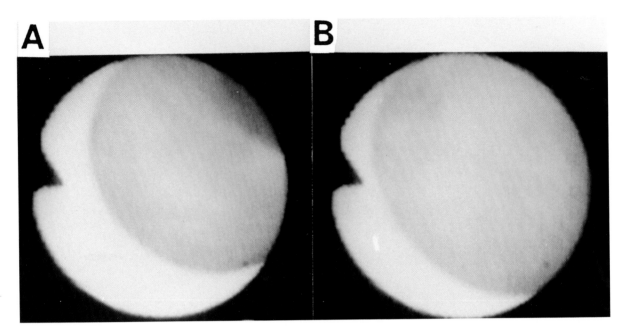

Fig. 7. The same wall segment 3 months later. **A:** during diastole. **B:** during systole. Note the pink color.

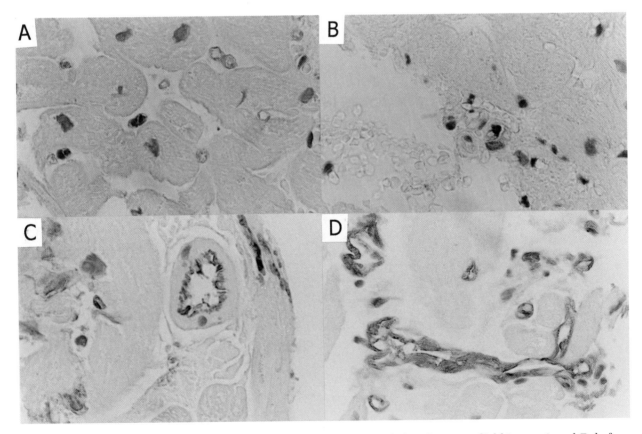

Fig. 8. Specimen obtained from the observed portion by cardioscope-guided endomyocardial biopsy. **A** and **B:** before angiogenic therapy. **C** and **D:** 3 months later. **A** and **C:** immunostain of factor 8 of endothelial cells. **B** and **D:** immunostain of alpha-actin of vascular smooth muscle cells. ×400.

References

1. Sarnoff SJ, Braunwald E, Welch GH Jr, et al: Hemodynamic determinants of oxygen consumption of the heart with special reference to the tension time index. Am J Physiol 192:148–156, 1958.
2. Oshima T, Hirose J, Sasaki T, et al: Candidates for angiogenic therapy. In: Studies on Angiogenic Therapy of Ischemic Heart Disease. Uchida Y (ed). Japan Circulation Society, 1996, pp 102–106 (in Japanese).
3. Yanagisawa-Miwa A, Uchida Y, Nakamura F, et al: Salvage of infarcted myocardium by angiogenic action of basic fibroblast growth factor. Science 257:1410–1413, 1992.
4. Uchida Y, Yanagisawa-Miwa A, Nakamura F, et al: Angiogenic therapy of acute myocardial infarction by intrapericardial injection of basic fibroblast growth factor and heparan sulfate. Am Heart J 130:1182–1188. 1995.
5. Uchida Y, Takeuchi K: Comparative studies on TMR and growth factors (VEGF and bFGF) for myocardial salvage. In: Studies on Angiogenic Therapy of Ischemic Heart Disease. Uchida Y (ed). Jpn Circulat Society, 1996, pp 83–91 (in Japanese).
6. Uchida Y, Nakamura F, Morita T, et al: Treatment of ASO with human recombinant bFGF. In: Studies on Angiogenic Therapy of Ischemic Heart Disease. Uchida Y (ed). Japan Circulation Society, 1996, pp 99–101 (in Japanese).

Chapter 29

Identification of Hibernating and Stunned Myocardium by Cardioscopy

Hibernating myocardium is temporarily asleep and can wake up to function normally when the blood supply is fully restored.[1] As shown in Chapter 28, pale wall segments without obvious contraction and white wall segments without atrophy and without contraction are considered hibernating myocardium, since contraction was restored upon restoration of blood flow.

Stunned myocardium is defined as that with reduced contraction but coronary blood flow is normal or increased[2] due to increased cytosolic calcium and formation of free radicals upon reperfusion.[3,4] However, exact cardioscopic features of stunned myocardium are not known.

Fig. 1 shows coronary angiograms before and 30 minutes after, and left ventriculograms 30 minutes after stent implantation into the right coronary artery in a patient with acute myocardial infarction. Stent implantation successfully recanalized the obstructed segment. However, ventricular contraction was not restored. Before stent implantation, the high posterior wall segment, akinetic by ventriculography, was light brown to light red by cardioscopy. Although contraction was not restored, the identical segment changed into red, indicating hyperemia (Fig. 2). Similar changes were observed in other patients (Table 1). Recovered blood flow without contraction improvement may indicate the existence of stunned myocardium.[1] Time course changes in such wall segments are not known.

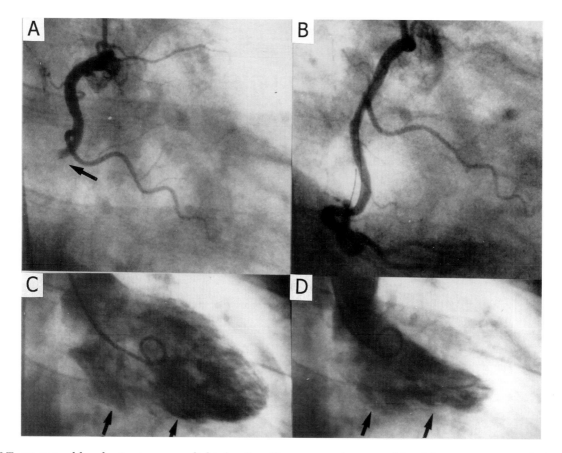

Fig. 1. M.T., 74-year-old male. Acute myocardial infarction. Coronary angiograms of the right coronary artery before (**A**) and 30 minutes after stent implantation to the middle segment of the artery. Left ventriculograms at end-diastole (**C**) and end-systole (**D**). Arrows: high posterior to inferior wall segments.

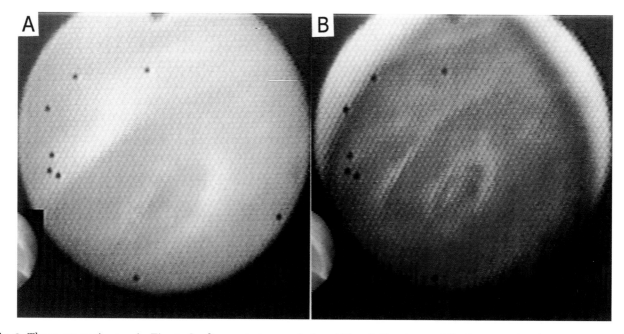

Fig. 2. The same patient as in Fig. 1. Cardioscopic images before (**A**) and 30 minutes (**B**) after stent implantation. Note the hyperemic endocardial surface after recanalization with stent implantation.

Table 1
**Changes in Endocardial Coloration Induced by Coronary
Interventions in Patients With Acute Myocardial Infarction**

	No. of Wall Segments	Color				Wall Motion		
		Light Brown	Pale	Purple	Red	Hypokinetic	Akinetic	Dyskinetic
1. Before intervention	10	1	5	4		2	6	2
2. After intervention	9			1	8		6	3

References

1. Rahimtoola SH: The hibernating myocardium. Am Heart J 117:211–221, 1989.
2. Braunwald F, Floner RA: The stunned myocardium: Prolonged postischemic ventricular dysfunction. Circulation 66:1146–1149, 1982.
3. Opie LH: Reperfusion injury and its pharmacological modification. Circulation 80:1049–1062, 1989.
4. Bolli R, Hartley CJ, Rahimtoola RS: Clinical relevance of myocardial "stunning." In: Stunning, Hibernation, and Calcium in Myocardial Ischemia and Reperfusion. Opie LH (ed). Kluwer Academic Publishers, Boston, 1992, pp 56–82.

PART III

Future Applications of Coronary Angioscopy and Cardioscopy

Chapter 30

New Modalities of
Coronary Angioscopy

Fluorescent Image Angioscopy for Discrimination of Cells and Substances Composing Coronary Vessels

By labeling the native cells with a fluorescent substance that has affinity to them, or by detecting their autofluorescence, the individual cells targeted for examination can be identified. This method can also be used for identification of substances in the vessel wall and myocardium.

Table 1 shows autofluorescence of several substances composing the vascular wall examined by fluorescence microscopy in vitro, suggesting that collagens, lipids, and calcium can be discriminated by comparing their autofluorescence.

When excited with an ultraviolet ray (350–385 nm) and collecting at 420 nm, the nonatherosclerotic human coronary artery exhibited blue color, indicating collagens were occupying the wall, while lipid deposited plaque exhibited yellow or orange colors. In the latter plaque, ceroids produced by macrophages were observed by microscopy in the same portion. The results suggest the possibility that macrophages that induce the plaques to be unstable can be detected by color fluorescent angioscopy. Also, by labeling with fluorescent agents, the existence of cells and substances targeted for examination can also be identified.

It is still difficult for the available color fluorescent angioscopes to discriminate the moving targets, such as coronary artery and cardiac chambers, due to insufficient sensitivity of color ICCD. Therefore, monochromatic fluorescent image angioscopy is still used in our catheterization laboratories.

Fig. 1 shows a fluorescent image of platelet aggregates labeled with fluorescein isothiocyanate conjugated (FITC) in a patient with acute myocardial infarction.

Simultaneous Observation of Coronary Artery by Angioscope and Intravascular Ultrasound (IVUS)

If coronary plaques are observed simultaneously by angioscope and IVUS, much more information on both the surface morphology and the structure of the plaque can be obtained.

Fig. 2 shows an angioscope and IVUS probe incorporated in a guiding balloon catheter for simultaneous observation of the vessel interior, and the images of the left main trunk (LMT) after Cavitron ultrasonic suction aspirator (CUSA) ablation of the plaque in a patient with stable angina pectoris. The exposed atheromatous layer was observed by angioscopy, and dilatation due to loss of intima was observed by IVUS. Since the use of this system is limited to the proximal coronary segments due to its large size, a smaller system for simultaneous observation of more distal coronary segments is under development in our laboratories.

255

Table 1
Autofluorescence of the Substances Composing the Human Coronary Artery

Excitation Wavelength (nm)	350–385	400–480	545–585
Collection Wavelength (nm)	420	515	610
Calcium	white	yellow	orange
Cholesterol	white	light yellow	orange
oxyLDL	light blue	yellow	orange
Lipoprotein a	white	light yellow	red
Collagen I	blue	green	dark yellow
Collagen II	light blue	green	red
Collagen III	bluish white	light green	dark orange
Collagen IV	white	light yellow	orange

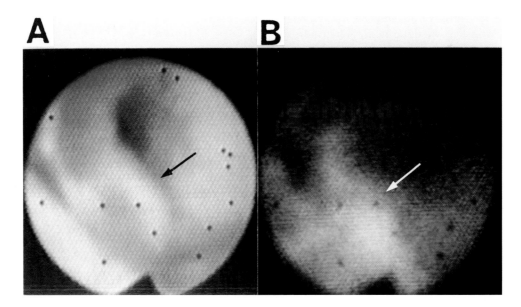

Fig. 1. S.T., 56-year-old male. Acute myocardial infarction. **A:** mixed thrombus by conventional angioscopy (arrow). **B:** fluorescence of platelet aggregates and fibrin labeled with FITC (arrow).

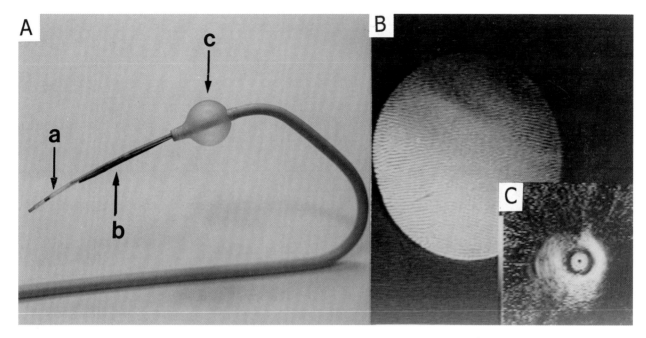

Fig. 2. M.T., 58-year-old male. Stable angina pectoris. **A:** a balloon guiding catheter incorporating a fiberscope and IVUS. **a:** IVUS. **b:** fiberscope. **c:** guiding balloon catheter. **B:** angioscopic image of LMT after CUSA. **C:** simultaneously obtained IVUS image of the same LMT.

Reference

1. Uchida Y: Atlas of Cardioangioscopy. Medical View Co., Tokyo, 1997.

Chapter 31

Angioscope-Guided Intracoronary Interventions

Angioscope-Guided Conventional Plain Old Balloon Angioplasty (POBA) and direct coronary atherectomy (DCA)

Intravascular ultrasound (IVUS)-guided angioplasty of coronary and peripheral arteries is now clinically used. However, angioscope-guided coronary angioplasty is still not established due to the large size of the equipment.

Fig. 1 shows various tools for angioscope-guided coronary interventions. By using these tools, processes of interventions can be observed.

Angioscope-Guided Mechanical Recanalization of Chronic Total Coronary Occlusion

Angioscope-guided balloon and laser angioscopy systems are routinely used for peripheral arteries in our laboratories;[1] however, they are not used for the coronary artery, due to difficulty in developing a thin system.

Fig. 1E shows a system for angioscope-guided mechanical recanalization of chronic total coronary occlusion. By using this system, even a long occlusive coronary segment can safely be opened. This system is now used for the peripheral artery in humans.

Angioscope-Guided Tissue Removal

Fig. 2A shows an angioscope-guided plaque remover for residual coronary plaques such as obstructive intimal flaps, which are frequently resistant to conventional angioplasty. Since this system is still large, its use is limited to removal of residual atherosclerotic plaques in the peripheral artery in our laboratories (Fig. 2B–D).

Angioscope-Guided Laser Coronary Angioplasty

Previously, laser coronary angioplasty was performed under fluoroscopic guidance. Therefore, coronary perforation occasionally occurred.[2] This serious complication is the major reason why laser coronary angioplasty is not widely used. If laser angioplasty is performed under angioscopic guidance, precise targeting can be attained and perforation can be prevented. Angioscope-guided laser angioplasty is restricted to the peripheral artery, solely due to the lack of a thin system. Fig. 3 shows an angioscope-guided laser angioplasty system that we devised. This system is essentially the same in structural size as the coronary angioscope now widely used in Japan, except there is a laser guide newly incorporated in it (see Chapter 2). This system is also feasible for photodynamic therapy of coronary plaques.[3]

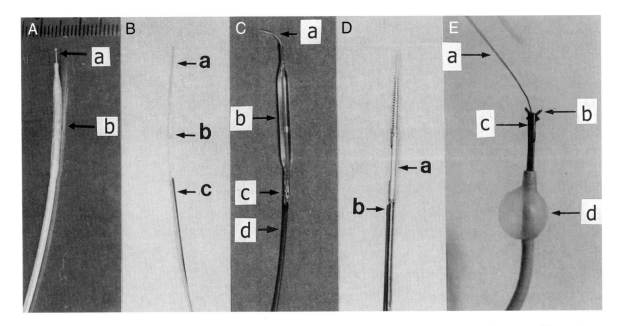

Fig. 1. Catheters with an attached angioscope for coronary interventions. **A:** balloon catheter with a steerable angioscope. **a:** 1.5 F fiberscope. **b:** balloon catheter. The fiberscope is exchangeable with a 1.014 guidewire. **B:** balloon catheter with a 1.5 F fiberscope fixed on it. **a:** guidewire. **b:** balloon catheter. **c:** 1.5 F fiberscope. **C:** IVUS-guided balloon catheter with a 1.5 F fiberscope for simultaneous guiding of POBA by IVUS and angioscopy. **a:** guidewire. **b:** balloon. **c:** IVUS. **d:** fiberscope. **D:** angioscope-guided DCA catheter. **a:** DCA catheter. **b:** 1.5 F fiberscope. **E:** angioscope-guided total occlusion opener. **a:** guidewire. **b:** cusps for opening. **c:** 1.5 F fiberscope. **d:** guiding balloon catheter.

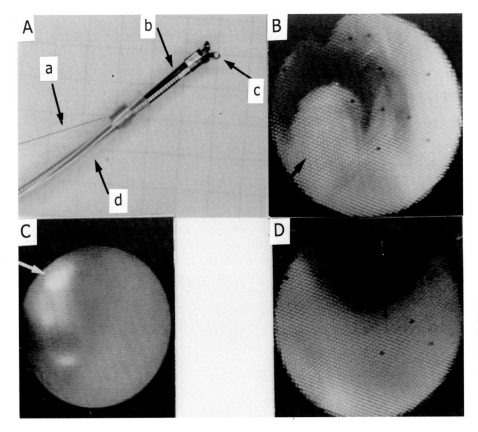

Fig. 2. A: angioscope-guided plaque remover. **a:** bending device. **b:** 1.5 F fiberscope. **c:** cusps for target removal. **d:** guiding catheter. A residual plaque in the superficial femoral artery in a patient with ASO before (**A**), during (**B**), and after removal (**C**). Arrow in A: residual plaque. Arrow in B: remover cusps.

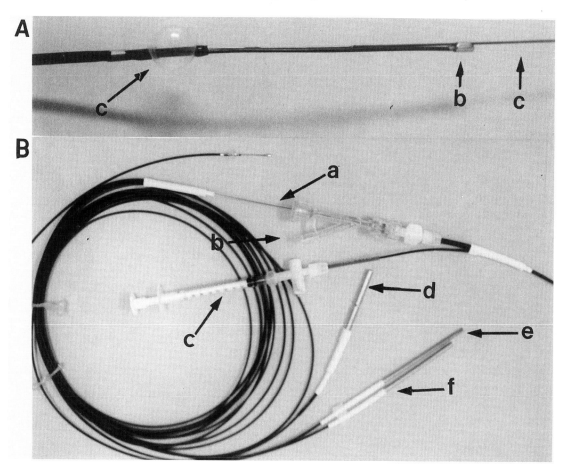

Fig. 3. Angioscope-guided laser coronary angioplasty catheter. **A:** distal part. **a:** guidewire. **b:** fiberscope part in which laser guide is incorporated. **c:** catheter part. **B:** proximal part. **a:** fiberscope controller. **b:** flush channel. **c:** balloon inflator. **d:** image guide. **e:** laser guide. **f:** light guide.

References

1. Uchida Y, Fujimori Y, Tomaru T, et al: Percutaneous angioplasty of chronic obstruction of peripheral arteries by a temperature-controlled Nd:YAG laser system in patients with arteriosclerosis obliterance. J Interven Cardiol 5:301–308, 1992.
2. Geschwind HJ, Tomaru T, Nakamura F, et al: Holmium YAD laser coronary angioplasty with multifiber catheters. J Interven Cardiol 4:171–179, 1991.
3. Katoh T, Asahara T, Naitoh Y, et al: In vivo intravascular laser photodynamic therapy in rabbit atherosclerotic lesions using a lateral direction fiber. Lasers Surg Med 20:373–381, 1997.

Chapter 32

Cardioscope-Guided Intracardiac Interventions

Cardioscope-Guided Intramyocardial Drug Administration for Treatment of Ischemic Heart Disease

The cardioscope-guided intramyocardial injection system is composed of a 27 G needle-tipped 3 F catheter, a 1.3 F fiberscope, and a 9 F guiding balloon catheter. The balloon is pushed against the cardiac luminal surface for cardioscopic observation. After confirmation of the target portion, the needle is inserted into the myocardium under cardioscopic guidance, and drugs are injected into the myocardium.

By this technique, ethanol was successfully injected into the canine ventricular septum. One month later, the septum was thin and fibrotic.[1] The ischemic portion of the myocardium can be identified by percutaneous cardioscopy. Therefore, cardioscope-guided intramyocardial injection of growth factors is a more accurate targeting angiogenic therapy of ischemic heart disease.[2]

Cardioscope-Guided Intrapericardial Therapy

About 15% of patients with ischemic heart disease are not indicated for interventional and surgical therapy and are not controlled with any available drugs. They are candidates for angiogenic therapy. However, the transarterial approach for this therapy is frequently difficult due to coronary and aortic anatomy and associated diseases. In these patients, intrapericardial administration through the right atrium is one curative therapy. Its feasibility was confirmed in an experimental canine model of acute myocardial infarction[3] and it is now clinically attempted in our laboratories.

References

1. Uchida Y, Nakamura F, Tomaru T, et al: Transcatheter treatment of HOCM: An experimental study. Jpn Circulat J 55(Suppl):98, 1991 (in Japanese).
2. Uchida Y, Takeuchi K: Comparative study on the angiogenic effects of transmyocardial laser revascularization and intramyocardial administration of growth factors. Report of Japan College of Circulation on Angiogenic Therapy of Ischemic Heart Disease, 1996, p 159 (in Japanese).
3. Uchida Y, Yanagisawa-Miwa, Nakamura F, et al: Angiogenic therapy of acute myocardial infarction by intrapericardial injection of basic fibroblast growth factor and heparan sulfate. Am Heart J 130:1182–1188, 1995.

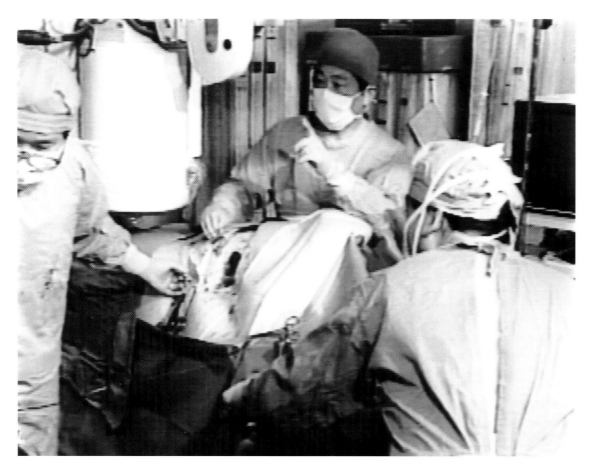

Dr. Yasumi Uchida.

INDEX

Page numbers that appear in *italics* indicate a figure or a table.